HEALTH MANUAL
A Self Help Guide

KT-102-695

A practical look-it-up-yourself book packed with reliable advice — invaluable for families, individuals, community health care.

It covers, in an accessible way, details about health maintenance, prevention of accidents and first aid, information about immunizations, advice about common tropical problems and how to avoid them — and what to do if you don't! — and a whole section on pregnancy and the first few months of life.

Four A–Z rapid reference sections give specific medical advice for men, women, adults and children and there is a glossary of some of the less common words often used by doctors and medical staff.

Dr Veronica Moss is a practising doctor as well as medical advisor to the Church Missionary Society. She has experience in obstetrics, child care, tropical medicine and community health care, and has worked in India, Ethiopia and Great Britain.

Health Manual

A SELF HELP GUIDE

DR VERONICA MOSS

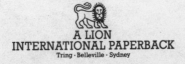

A LION
INTERNATIONAL PAPERBACK
Tring · Belleville · Sydney

Copyright © 1986 Veronica Moss

Published by
Lion Publishing plc
Icknield Way, Tring, Herts, England
ISBN 0 85648 919 0
Lion Publishing Corporation
10885 Textile Road, Belleville, Michigan 48111, USA
ISBN 0 85648 919 0
Albatross Books Pty Ltd
PO Box 320, Sutherland, NSW 2232, Australia
ISBN 0 86760 647 9

First edition 1986
Reprinted 1986

Every effort has been made to ensure that the
advice given in this book is correct and in line with
good medical practice. The author and publishers
cannot accept liability for any problems which may
arise as a result of using this book.

All rights reserved

British Library Cataloguing in Publication Data

Moss, Veronica
    Health manual.—(A Lion international paperback)
    1. Self-care, Health—Social aspects
    I. Title
    613   RA776.95
    ISBN 0 85648 919 0

Printed and bound in Great Britain by
Cox and Wyman, Reading

Contents

INTRODUCTION

The purpose of this book

- What can I do for myself if I'm ill?
- When is it important to seek medical help?
- What if my child is ill?
- What can I do to maintain my health and the health of my children?
- What can I do to prevent illness?

There are millions of people who do not have easy access to a doctor or for whom the cost of seeking medical advice may be a real problem. For others a doctor or medical advice may be instantly available at the end of a telephone, or an ambulance can be called out within minutes of an emergency. Even so, people often hesitate and wonder what they could be doing for themselves instead. Many feel it is important that we learn to rely on ourselves, that we do not become entirely dependent on the medical help just around the corner, and that we do not take drugs and medicines as the only answer to life's problems.

This book seeks to meet all these needs.

Health and wholeness

The search for health and wholeness occupies much of many people's lives today. In some countries there is a popular movement away from the straight scientific application of western or 'allopathic' medicine. This has tended to see health and illness in terms of cause and effect, often isolating episodes of illness from the whole personality of the patient and his or her circumstances.

Today there is a growing search for a wholeness of approach, taking into full account the needs of the body, the mind and the spirit, and seeing illness as a result of a dis-integration between these aspects of a human being. Of course, a person's external circumstances do affect health — but reactions to those circumstances are also very important to the progress or otherwise of disease. If people have been made in the image of God, this means, among other things, that we have a body through which the mind and the spirit are expressed; each has to be given its proper place of importance. The needs of each have to be catered for in the search for wholeness and health.

Full integration of mind and spirit leads us to wholeness. Integration can be achieved by following the way we have been designed to work. If we are the result of creation, not random accident, we would expect the Creator, the Designer, to have a basic plan for us. So wholeness ultimately involves our relationship with God as it is explained in the Bible. But much of his basic plan and design is also obvious in nature. Dis-integration is the result of going against that plan. It is like a car: sooner or later it will grind to a halt if the manufacturer's instructions are ignored.

Our bodies have an in-built tendency towards healing. They have a wonderful defence system against invading foreign bodies such as bacteria and viruses. It is, of course, not foolproof — as we all know. Doctors, 'healers' and healthworkers of any sort do not heal — what they do is try to promote the drive the body already has towards healing by removing obstacles to that healing. For instance, a wound needs to be cleansed of debris and dirt, and the surface to be protected against invasion by bacteria, to allow the body to heal itself.

Some medicines will strengthen the natural drive towards healing, and may be needed to overcome the forces that are tending towards 'dis-integration' or illness. But the body's own resources can be maintained and improved by correct nutrition, adequate rest, relaxation and sleep, sufficient exercise and attention given to mental and spiritual needs.

We all know that death is part of human existence, that our lives and our resources are limited, and that illness of some sort, or the final failure of our bodies, will bring our bodies to an end. But life does not end there. Preparation for death and the life hereafter should also be part of living, and of the search for wholeness.

Our relationships with others, our families and communities, and on a larger scale with our nation and people of other nationalities, races and creeds, are also of utmost importance in this search for personal wholeness. Living at peace within our communities, with neighbours and other nationalities could lead to a wholeness and integration of the human race, to a true 'brotherhood of man' — but there has first to be a peace and harmony within ourselves and in our relationship with God before this wider harmony is possible.

WHERE DOES IT HURT?

Look at the simple diagram below. Decide where your pain is on the body. Look up the general headings related to that area in the index. Then turn to the relevant pages in the rapid reference section.

If the problem is the kind only experienced by men or by women, turn to the special section that deals with these. Remember that there is also a special section for children.

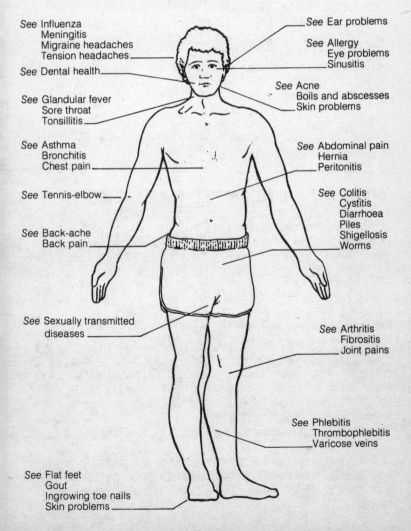

See Influenza
Meningitis
Migraine headaches
Tension headaches
See Dental health

See Glandular fever
Sore throat
Tonsillitis

See Asthma
Bronchitis
Chest pain

See Tennis-elbow

See Back-ache
Back pain

See Sexually transmitted
diseases

See Flat feet
Gout
Ingrowing toe nails
Skin problems

See Ear problems

See Allergy
Eye problems
Sinusitis

See Acne
Boils and abscesses
Skin problems

See Abdominal pain
Hernia
Peritonitis

See Colitis
Cystitis
Diarrhoea
Piles
Shigellosis
Worms

See Arthritis
Fibrositis
Joint pains

See Phlebitis
Thrombophlebitis
Varicose veins

1 HEALTH MAINTENANCE

1.1 Nutrition

Our bodies are 'built' by the foods we eat. Foods are broken down in our digestive system into smaller components which can be absorbed into the bloodstream. They are then carried to different parts of our bodies.

At the different 'sites', the particular 'building blocks' which are needed for growth, maintenance or healing are taken out of the bloodstream to be used in the cells and tissues. It is therefore very important to provide the body with the foods that contain the right 'building blocks'. To do this we need to understand the meaning of a 'balanced diet'. This is made up of:

- body-building foods (proteins)
- energy foods (carbohydrates)
- energy storage and some building materials (fats)
- protective foods (vitamins and minerals)
- fibre

TO PLAN A BALANCED DAILY DIET

For a healthy diet, include a few foods from each of the 4 groups listed. For more details, see the charts in this section.

In practice, the simplest way to plan a balanced meal is to plan the main meal of the day around a protein food. Add a good helping of fresh vegetables with potatoes, bread or rice, and start or end with some fresh fruit if possible. Get to know which foods contain iron (an essential part of the blood) and calcium (for teeth, bones, muscle and other body tissues).

If you are unable to eat meat, there is no need to fear that you are not getting a balanced diet. If you choose something from each group of foods during the day, you will probably be eating enough to keep you reasonably healthy. Make up for the lack of meat or fish by eating more from group 4, the dairy foods, if you can. If you cannot eat those either, then it is more important to know the other groups well and to 'mix and match' them as well as possible, and to increase the amount of nuts and beans that you eat.

This section contains a brief explanation about protein foods; how to ensure that you have an adequate intake of these important 'building-blocks'; and a brief introduction to the other foods.

GROUP 1
Fruit and vegetables

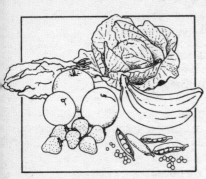

The main source of vitamins, but also provide sugars, fibre, iron and calcium (green leafy vegetables).

GROUP 2
Carbohydrates in starchy foods, cereals and root vegetables

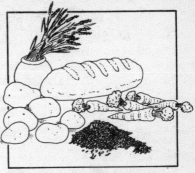

These provide starch and sugars (which are turned into fuel for energy in our bodies) and fibre, as well as protein and some iron and calcium.

GROUP 3
Proteins in meat and alternatives

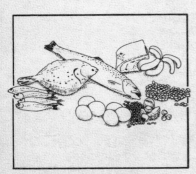

Eat fish, beans, nuts, lentils or eggs as alternatives to meat. They also provide iron; fish provide calcium and nuts provide fats.

GROUP 4
Proteins and fats in dairy products

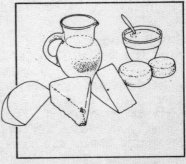

Eat milk, yoghurt or cheese to provide calcium for bones and teeth as well as good proteins.

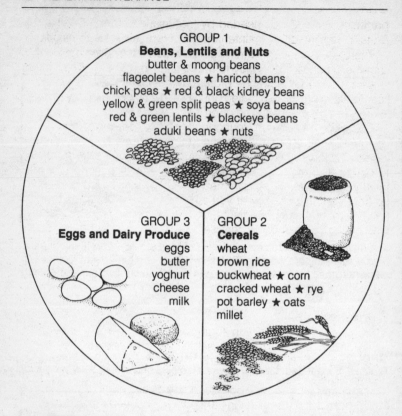

GROUP 1
Beans, Lentils and Nuts
butter & moong beans
flageolet beans ★ haricot beans
chick peas ★ red & black kidney beans
yellow & green split peas ★ soya beans
red & green lentils ★ blackeye beans
aduki beans ★ nuts

GROUP 3
Eggs and Dairy Produce
eggs
butter
yoghurt
cheese
milk

GROUP 2
Cereals
wheat
brown rice
buckwheat ★ corn
cracked wheat ★ rye
pot barley ★ oats
millet

Protein foods

When digested, protein foods are broken down into amino acids. These are the basic 'building-blocks' from which an amazing variety of proteins can be re-made in our bodies — rather like the letters of the alphabet can be made into an infinite variety of words and sentences.

Amino acids are the basic 'bricks' from which our bodies are constructed. But just as a house cannot be constructed from bricks or stones only but needs cement or binding material to hold it together (and other refinements like internal plastering, wiring and plumbing to make it comfortable) so our bodies also require fats, starches, vitamins and minerals to complete the 'building'.

Amino acids have to be combined in a variety of ways to make different structures and tissues. As they are carried around in the bloodstream, the different tissues 'pick' or select out the particular amino acids needed by that tissue to form its own proteins for growth or maintenance.

There are 8 essential amino acids which have to be eaten together to enable the body to make full use of them. When these 8 are found together in one protein, that food is known as a 'complete protein'; it is called 'incomplete' when only some of them are found in one type of protein.

Complete proteins are found in meat, fish, eggs and dairy products; incomplete proteins are found in vegetables, nuts and cereals. The incomplete proteins can be put together in such a way that all 8 amino acids will be provided in one meal. This will give you a complete protein meal even if you have not been able to eat meat, fish or eggs. If you add milk, cheese or eggs to a meal without these ingredients, you can be even more sure that you have provided some complete proteins for the body to use.

The diagram shows the 3 main groups of non-meat proteins. If you choose foods from each segment and put them together in any one meal, you will have provided your body with a complete set of the essential amino acids.

Carbohydrates

Carbohydrates are found in sugar and starch (cereals, fruit and root vegetables) and are an essential part of our diet. They are necessary to give our bodies energy. However, eating too much refined sugar (found in white and brown sugar, honey, syrup and sweets) can lead to a person becoming overweight.

Carbohydrates provide 'instant energy' because they can be sent more or less straight into the bloodstream as fuel for energy. They are used up quickly, or if not used at once, turned into fat and stored.

The sugars contained in fruit and in unrefined cereal foods take longer to break down into usable sugars. This is partly because of the high fibre content. Fibre itself is not digested so there is a slower, more sustained release of the energy-giving nutrient into the bloodstream. This is particularly important to remember for people who are diabetic. A diet that relies on fruit, unrefined cereals and root vegetables for its supply of carbohydrates may even help to prevent the onset of the adult type of diabetes. Those who need to lose weight also benefit from this diet: it is more filling and leaves you feeling less hungry.

Fats

Weight for weight, fats are the foods that contain the highest levels of energy, because they provide many calories per gram.

The body needs fats for the structure of tissues such as nerves and also for helping to regulate the blood-clotting mechanism. But only a small amount (about 30gm, just over an ounce) is needed each day.

There are animal (or saturated) fats and vegetable (polyunsaturated) fats. There is some evidence that the vegetable fats are, on the whole, more healthy for us than animal fats, most of which are high in cholesterol. Small amounts of animal fats are important, but should not be our only source of fats. High levels of cholesterol in the blood are associated with heart disease and high blood pressure, and people who eat a lot of any type of fat are often overweight.

Animal fats are found in meat, especially pork, lamb, sausages and tinned meats, and in dairy products such as butter, cream, and whole milk; egg yolks contain a lot of cholesterol and 3–4 eggs per week is probably the maximum number you should eat unless eggs are your only source of complete proteins.

Vegetable fats are found in nuts, soya beans, sunflower and mustard seeds, among others, and margarines and cooking oils are usually made from these sources.

Those who need to lose weight should remember that cooking will alter the fat content of the foods you eat. Frying or roasting foods will increase their fat level considerably, while boiling or grilling them will reduce it.

Fibre

It is believed that a lack of fibre in our diets encourages the development of diseases such as chronic constipation, piles (haemorrhoids), varicose veins, and perhaps deep vein thrombosis, diverticulitis, and possibly even cancer of the colon. It is also thought that diabetes, obesity, some heart diseases and raised blood pressure may be associated with a low-fibre diet.

There is still much research needed on this subject, but in the mean-time, there is no doubt that a high fibre diet tends to improve constipation and some other bowel problems. It reduces the amount of cholesterol being absorbed from the gut and slows down the entry of sugars into the bloodstream. A high fibre diet is therefore being recommended by doctors to treat or prevent quite a number of diseases, including obesity and diabetes. It is a very good diet for those who need to lose weight as it is filling, makes you less hungry for longer and is probably much healthier than crash diets or special slimming diets tried by thousands of people all over the world without much lasting success.

Vitamins and minerals

Most of the protein foods, vegetables and fruit are rich in vitamins and minerals. They are essential to life, growth and reproduction. Details of these are given in the following charts.

1. Sources of important vitamins

Vitamins	Rec. daily intake	Main function	Main sources
*Vitamin A (Retinol)	0.75mg	Forms part of the eye and its pigment. Helps to maintain mucus membranes. (Early sign of deficiency is 'night blindness'.)	Green leafy vegetables, red and orange/yellow fruit and vegetables; milk, butter, cheese, eggs, cod liver oil, liver, enriched margarines.
Vitamin B1 (Thiamin)	1.2mg	Together with B2 and nicotinic acid, helps to release energy from foods.	Wholegrain cereals, lentils, peas, beans and nuts; liver, kidney, and milk.
Vitamin B2 (Riboflavin)	1.7mg		
Nicotinic acid	1.8mg		
Vitamin B6 (Pyridoxine)	2mg	Involved in various body functions including production of antibodies, and some brain biochemicals. (Deficiency in some women causes premenstrual problems — increase dose to 50–100mg daily.)	Meat, liver, kidney, milk, eggs, nuts, high fibre cereals, some vegetables and yeast.
Vitamin B12 (Cyanocobalamin)	0.001mg	Essential for production and maintenance of body cells including red blood cells.	Meat, liver, dairy products. Not present in plant foods.

1. Sources of important vitamins

Folic acid		Essential for the formation of body cells: production and maintenance of red blood cells in particular.	Liver, beans, peas, nuts, green vegetables and wholegrain cereals.
Choline		General body maintenance.	Egg yolk, liver, wholegrain cereals, beans, peas and nuts.
Pantothenic acid		General body maintenance.	Present in most foods.
Vitamin C (Ascorbic acid)	30mg	General body maintenance. Promotes healing processes. Some people believe it protects against virus and bacterial infections.	Citrus and other fruits, green vegetables, potatoes and tomatoes.
*Vitamin D (Cholecalciferol)	0.003mg	Essential for bone growth and maintenance working together with calcium.	Sunlight on skin causes production of vitamin D. Also present in fish liver oil, dairy products and enriched margarine, and in some fish.
*Vitamin E (Tochopherols)	10mg	Appears to be involved in variety of cell functions.	Seeds and nuts, enriched margarines and green leafy vegetables.

1. Sources of important vitamins

*Vitamin K (K_1 and K_2)	These are an essential part of the blood-clotting mechanism.	Absorption from gut where bacteria synthesize it; green leafy vegetables, wholegrain cereals, fruits and nuts. (Breast-fed babies are often given an injection of this in the first few days of life as breast milk is not a good source and they have not yet acquired intestinal bacteria.

*Fat-soluble vitamins

2. Sources of important minerals

Mineral	Main function	Main sources
Calcium and phosphorous	Essential for bones and teeth, growth and maintenance. Also for blood clotting, muscle and nerve activity, and energy transfer.	Green vegetables, cereals, fish, meat and milk.
Sodium	Maintenance of body fluids. High levels may be associated with raised blood pressure.	Present in most foods and in table salt.
Potassium	Similar functions to sodium.	Fruit and fruit juices (including bananas), cereals and in many other foods.
Iron	Essential for blood formation (the oxygen-carrying part, haemoglobin).	Green leafy vegetables, green vegetables, apricots and prunes, wholegrain cereals, meat, kidney and liver.

2. Sources of important minerals

Fluoride	Important for protection of surface of teeth against decay.	Drinking water, tea, fluoride toothpastes. (Beware of high levels in water supplies: overdose causes discolouration of teeth and other problems.)
Iodine	Needed for formation of thyroxine, a hormone regulating the metabolism.	Fish liver oils and sea foods, iodized salts.

There are many other minerals and trace elements that are required in minute quantities, but most are present in the common foods.

3. Sources of carbohydrates, sugar and fibre

Unrefined high fibre

Fruit — dried and fresh
Nuts (preferably with skins)
Cereals — wholemeal flour and
bread
— brown rice
— oats
— barley, rye etc.
and anything made with the above
Beans
Root vegetables
— including potatoes with their
skins, yams and cassava
(cassava leaves contain more
protein, fibre and vitamins than
the root, and both can be eaten
together)

Refined low fibre

Sweets and chocolates
Fizzy drinks and squashes
Sweet biscuits and cakes (made
with white flour)
White bread
Jam, honey, marmalade
Puddings and desserts made
from the above
Instant packet soups and sauces

Crisps, savoury biscuits and
snacks made from white flour or
potatoes

SPECIAL HINTS FOR A HEALTHY DIET

For weightwatchers
Eat a diet of
● high fibre ● low sugar ● low fat
and limit your calories to 1,000–1,500 per day if you want to lose weight. This is also a good diet for diabetics or those with diabetes in the family.

For those with high blood pressure

If high blood pressure runs in your family, it is also advisable to follow this diet.

Eat a diet of
- high fibre
- low sugar
- low fat (especially cholesterol)
- low salt (salt substitutes do not help: avoid them too)

Most people in colder climates eat more salt than needed. Salt is present in most foods and it is not usually necessary to add any to have an adequate intake.

NOTE

If you live in a hot climate and you perspire a lot, you may need more salt as you lose it in sweat.

For those with little money to spend

Remember
- Breast milk is — cheap
  - clean
  - safe
  - provides all the baby needs for growth for at least 5 – 6 months
  - provides some protection against infection.
- Eggs are a good, usually cheap, source of protein for growth.
- Chicken (cooked to be tender and cut up into very small pieces for babies over 6 months) is also a good source of protein for growth.
- Fish is an excellent source of protein, and is often quite cheap. It also contains some vitamins and minerals, and much of the fat is poly-unsaturated, thus helping to reduce the risk of developing raised blood pressure or heart problems.
- Liver, kidneys and other offal are usually cheaper than meat and have high protein, iron and vitamin contents.
- Beans, peas, lentils and nuts are a very cheap and good source of protein.
- Green leafy vegetables, including the leaves of sweet potatoes, beans, peas, pumpkins, squash and baobab have some protein and iron, and much vitamin A.
- Cassava leaves (especially young leaves), soaked and thoroughly prepared, can be eaten with the root: they have more protein and provide more vitamins.
- Yellow and red fruits and vegetables, including pawpaws (which also contain protein) and tomatoes, are a good source of vitamin A.

If you are concerned that your child is not getting enough to eat, then look at these 3 things to assess if this is true:

● Does he have lots of energy and enjoyment?
● Is he putting on weight, even if it is only slowly (weigh once a month)?
● Is he growing in height (measure and mark on a wall or chart each month)?

If the answer is yes, then you do not need to worry. If the answer is no, then you should take your child for a check-up by a doctor or a trained nurse.

1.2 Exercise

CHILDREN

Exercise is good at any age. Healthy children are full of energy and run around playing or exploring all the time: they will soon stop when they run out of energy.

ADULTS

Adults also need exercise, but tend to take less as they grow older. Some exercise may be part of your job, but if not, then it is more important that you do some regular exercise each week. Walking 2–3 miles a day, swimming or games are very good exercise.

Some people prefer to do specific exercises at home, or to dance to music. What you do is not as important as the fact that you take some exercise. It is also important to build up any kind of exercise gradually: do not start suddenly trying to do a lot if you have been doing nothing for months or years. Start by going for a walk or a short jog, or by doing a 10 minute exercise session at home every day; then gradually increase the amount you do over a period of weeks. Remember that muscles that have not been used much for months will protest at first by becoming sore and achy for a few days. You must continue the exercise to 'work through' that and accustom your muscles to the extra work.

1.3 Stress

Stress is usually talked about as if it is a bad thing. This is not true. Stress can be good or bad. We all need some challenge or stimulus to produce good results, to work hard and achieve something, and this can be counted as good, useful stress. Stress becomes bad when it begins to result in tension, anxiety and poorer results: in other words, when it becomes unproductive.

We need to know ourselves well enough to recognize when stress is becoming bad for us, or when our reactions to the stress are causing problems. It may be the stress itself that needs to be stopped or changed; it may be our reactions to the stress. Stress that is prolonged, unrelieved and which leads to constant tension can eventually result in the sort of situation shown in the diagram.

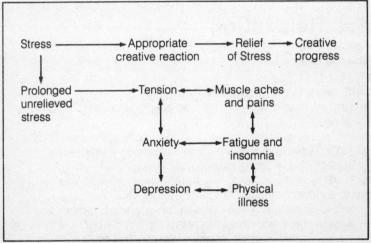

When we react by being tense or anxious about a situation, our muscles 'tense up'. The first to tense tend to be the shoulder and neck muscles, and sometimes the stomach muscles. When these muscles remain tense for a while we may become aware of a tension headache developing. This feels like a steel band around the head, caused by the shoulder muscles pulling on the scalp which in turn becomes sore and tense. Others experience a 'knot' in the stomach when their 'middle' feels sore or tight. This may be accompanied by some burning discomfort because, in some people, the stomach lining is also affected by tension. If you are aware that these feelings or pains are becoming quite common for you, try to do the following:

● Take a good look at the source of the stress: is there anything you can do about it? Can the stress be reduced? Can you discuss it with anyone?
● Take a good look at yourself: why are you reacting as you are? Could you change your own reaction? Do you have to become tense, angry, frustrated? Do you have to worry so much? Discuss it with someone.

- If none of these solutions are possible take a good look at what you *can* do: can you take a break? Can you take some time away from the stressful situation? Learn techniques of muscle and mind relaxation and apply them regularly. For some people, vigorous exercise will relieve feelings of tension. Find out what works for you.

For a more detailed discussion of this subject see *Anxiety and Tension* and *Depression*, section 5.1.

1.4 Relaxation

There are many techniques for relaxation. One technique is outlined here.

One relaxation technique

- Find yourself a warm, quiet and comfortable spot to sit or lie down.
- You might like some quiet soothing music in the background.
- Take a couple of deep breaths in and out, then breathe quietly, slowly and gently.
- Starting with your toes, first tighten every muscle you can think of, and then let it go completely. Work your way up each leg and arm, including your bottom, back and abdomen, and so to neck, face and scalp. If you find a muscle tightens again as you are relaxing other muscles, tighten and relax it again, then try to forget it and work on upwards. End by allowing your whole body to relax, sinking into the bed or chair and remain like that, breathing quietly and gently, for 10-15 minutes. Some people experience a floating sensation.
- Some find they can pray or meditate quietly during this exercise.

1.5 Sleep

We all need sleep — but some need it for longer periods than others. Most babies sleep a great deal of the time: sometimes in short naps; sometimes for several hours, with hours of wakefulness between — a baby's pattern does not usually conform to the parents'! But we each have our own pattern in adult life too, and again, some need more sleep than others.

If you are lucky enough to need only a few hours, with perhaps a 10 minute 'cat-nap' during the day, be thankful: you can be very usefully productive during hours when others are fast asleep! There is no need to resort to sleeping tablets to make sure you sleep as much as the expected 7 – 8 hours 'norm'. If you are not more tired the next day and your work is not affected, try to use the extra time happily instead. If you *do* find your work affected then you may need to discuss it with someone, perhaps a doctor, who can advise you.

If your sleep is affected by stress or worry, then try the suggestions in the section on stress. In particular, try to learn some muscle and mind relaxation techniques (see *Relaxation*, section 1.4) and apply them before going to bed, and perhaps while lying in bed, too, instead of counting sheep or worrying that you cannot sleep! You may need to talk about the worry with someone when it is possible or convenient.

If you cannot sleep
● Try to sort out the stress and your reaction to it.
● Apply relaxation techniques.
● Listen to music, or read a book (not one that is too gripping!).
● Make a hot drink and have a snack: this sometimes induces sleepiness (as well as, for some unfortunates, a weight problem).

1.6 Drugs and medicines
Drugs are any substances contained in tablets, liquid mixtures, injections or suppositories which, when used properly and in the right dosages, are health-promoting, but which, when used wrongly and in over-dosage, are harmful. The term 'medicine' is often used to mean only drugs in liquid form, and the term 'drugs' is often, now, used only to mean the 'heavy', addictive sort. Here these words will be used interchangeably and with their wider meaning.

DRUGS WHICH CAN CAUSE ADDICTION OR DEPENDENCE
You can become emotionally dependent on aspirin or cups of tea or coffee. You become physically dependent on a drug when it becomes incorporated into your body metabolism in such a way that to stop taking it produces physical reactions which can only be relieved by topping up with more of the same drug. For example, in regular excessive coffee or tea drinkers, a day without either might result in a severe headache. (Two or 3 cups of coffee in a day should be the maximum: one cup of strong coffee contains the therapeutic dose of caffeine.) Smokers are

physically addicted to nicotine, as well as emotionally dependent on the feel of the cigarette or pipe in their hands or on their lips. Emotional dependence may become a problem in itself, but emotional and physical dependence tends to lead on to true addiction. Here the body comes to 'need' the drug to function, but is sooner or later damaged by it, as in alcoholism or addiction to some of the tranquillizers and strong pain-killers.

NON-ADDICTIVE ESSENTIAL DRUGS FOR LONG-TERM USE

There are many drugs which the body 'needs' for entirely different reasons. A diabetic, for example, needs insulin to live because his own production of insulin has ceased, or a person with high blood pressure needs medication to prevent damage to blood-vessels, a stroke or a heart attack. There are some who need vitamin B12 injections to prevent a particular type of anaemia developing and others who need anti-depressants for longer or shorter times. None of these things come into the category of addiction and should be taken if prescribed by a doctor, without qualms about 'becoming dependent'. Your body is already dependent on them to survive, and the drugs are simply doing something your body would normally be doing itself.

DRUGS FOR SPECIFIC EPISODES AND EMERGENCIES

There is a large group of other medicines which come into neither of these categories, and used wisely, preferably under medical supervision, can be life-saving and extremely useful in controlling problems such as pain, asthma, hay fever and infections. See *Antibiotics*, section 8, *Asthma*, section 5.1.

IF YOU DO NOT HAVE ACCESS TO A DOCTOR:

- Get to know a small number of useful drugs for emergency use and stick to them.
- Be very careful to follow instructions about dosage and **never** take more.
- Use them only for **known** problems.
- Never take anything for more than the emergency situation without consulting a doctor (unless already instructed about long-term use).

- Always find out **what** the medicine is that you are being given and make a note of the name. This may be very valuable information for any doctor who later has to take over future treatment.
- Check the expiry date of any drugs (including creams and ointments) you buy.
- See the check list of useful medicines in section 8.

IS IT POSSIBLE TO AVOID CANCER?

There are a lot of things we can do to minimize the risks of developing cancer, even if we cannot be sure of avoiding it. Early detection and treatment helps as some forms of cancer can be cured.

This list of basic rules will help to minimize the risks and help to maintain general health.

- Do not smoke cigarettes, pipes or cigars.
- Drink alcohol only in moderation, if at all.
- Take care not to expose yourself too intensely to the sun or to ultraviolet lamps.
- Avoid asbestos dust.
- Use barrier methods of contraception (if avoidance of pregnancy is not of absolute importance) — they seem to help prevent cancer of the cervix — and have a regular smear test done.
- Avoid obesity and maintain a healthy diet by:
  — cutting down on fatty foods
  — eating plenty of fibre
  — eating plenty of fresh fruit and vegetables
- Observe safety regulations at work.
- Women should examine their breasts regularly (1–3 monthly): if there is any persistent lump or change, see a doctor as soon as possible.

2 PREVENTION AND FIRST AID

2.1 First-aid kit

It is useful to keep a box stocked with all or most of the following items. Keep the box locked and out of reach of children. This list includes suggestions of what to take with you if you are travelling, particularly to a tropical country.

General
- assorted sticking plasters (reputable brand)
- sterile gauze
- cotton wool
- crépe bandages — wide and narrow
- triangular bandage/sling
- safety pins
- scissors
- sterilized needle and tweezers for removing splinters
- witch-hazel for bruises and sprains
- antiseptic such as Savlon, Cetavlon, TCP or Dettol
- calamine lotion or cream (for sunburn or prickly heat)
- suntan lotion: high protection factor (5 or more) if you burn easily or are experiencing strong sun for the first time
- a small electric coil to use in a jug or glass to boil water prior to drinking or brushing teeth
- antibiotic powder, such as Cicatrin (available on prescription only in some countries)
- eye bath
- Mycil or Tinaderm cream and powder for those prone to fungal infections
- Bonjela for mouth ulcers and teething children
- a medicine measure, or 5ml teaspoon
- a thermometer

Tablets
- aspirin or paracetamol tablets, for headaches, odd aches and pains
- throat lozenges, such as Merocets, Vicks or Dequadin
- for diarrhoea, a choice of the following to control symptoms: codeine phosphate 30mg, 1–2 tabs 3 times per day (will constipate if taken for more than a couple of days); Imodium capsules, 2 at once, 1 after each stool to a maximum of 8 in 24 hours; Lomotil, 2 at once, 1 every 6 hours until diarrhoea stops; Kaolin mixture. These will **not** cure, but are useful if you are travelling. **Always replace fluid loss**.
See *Diarrhoea*, section 5.1

- Marzine, Avomine, Kwells, Sea Legs or Stugeron for those prone to travel sickness: all but Stugeron will make you drowsy and should not be taken with alcohol
- Piriton tablets for those who have any known allergies
- (Piriton 10mg for injection, with needle and syringe, for those with severe known allergies, to be available for a doctor or nurse to give if necessary)
- Rennies or similar for those prone to indigestion
- anti-malarials for prevention, plus Chloroquine tablets for an attack (complete course equals 12 tablets) (See section 6 for full discussion of malaria)
- sterilizing tablets for emergency water purification
- cough mixture, such as Codeine, Actifed Compound (see *Coughs and colds*, section 5.1): effective cough suppressants cause constipation and drowsiness
- a decongestant, such as Ephedrine nasal drops or an inhalant, such as Karvol, Vick, Friar's Balsam, menthol or eucalyptus oils
- an adequate supply of your regular medication, including the contraceptive Pill

---

NOTE
If you live in or are travelling to an area where there are no medicines available there is a list of antibiotics and other useful medicines, with dosages and advice about their use in section 8. Buy a small supply of essential medicines when you visit a larger centre or before you travel.

NOTE
For information on how to use a thermometer or how to take a pulse, see pages 259–60.

2.2 Accidents
PREVENTION — IN THE HOME

Poison and medicines
- Keep out of reach of children, high up or locked away.
- Do not keep poisons such as insecticides or petrol in soft drink bottles. If you **must**, keep them high up, out of reach of children, and **label** them!

Fires and cookers
- Keep children away, unless there is a supervised cooking session in progress!

Electricity
- Beware of electrocuting yourself or getting a severe shock when handling faulty sockets: wear rubber-soled shoes and rubber gloves if you have to handle any electric wiring or sockets, and turn off the electricity at the mains supply before doing any repairs.
- Train toddlers not to poke fingers or objects into sockets, or to play with leads or plugs.
- Child-proof sockets are available in some countries.

Indoors
- Use a stepladder or some other firm base when changing light bulbs, or reaching for things on high shelves.
- Do not have worn rugs, rugs on slippery floors, or ill-fitting shoes that can cause you to trip.

Outdoors
- Do not allow children to run around bare-foot because of the danger of dirty nails and thorns and, in some countries, snakes, scorpions and hookworms.

Ditches, wells and ponds
- Deep ditches should be fenced, wells should be covered and children should always be supervised while swimming, even in small, shallow ponds. Beware of rubbish pits where tins, glass and other sharp objects are thrown. Wrap such objects yourself in layers of newspaper before throwing them out.

PREVENTION — ON THE ROAD

Maintenance
- Ensure your vehicle is regularly serviced.
- All tyres, including the spare wheel, should be at the correct pressure and in good condition, with a good tread over the whole tyre surface and no cuts or bulges.

- Brakes and lights should be checked frequently.
- Jack, fuses and other essential equipment should be taken on every journey.

Seat belts
- Should be worn by driver and front seat passenger for all journeys, however short.
- Have belts comfortably firm.
- Children should travel on rear seats and some form of restraint safety seat or harness should be used. If this is not possible, an adult should sit with the child in the back.

Other drivers
- Keep alert for unpredictable drivers: not all drivers are as sensible and safe as you are! Even when they are, a sudden tyre 'blow-out' may occur, or an animal or child run across the road.

Wet, muddy roads
- Drive slowly, and check your brakes after going through water.

Yourself
- Don't drive if you feel ill or tired.
- Never drive if you have taken alcohol or such medications as sleeping tablets, tranquillizers, 'cold cures', or anti-histamines.

Motor-cyclists
- You and your pillion passenger should both wear crash helmets.
- Long sleeves and jeans, for protection against minor abrasions, are advisable, as are fluorescent clothing and gloves.

Break-downs or accidents
- Be prepared by always carrying a first-aid kit, torch, a few tools and emergency rations such as some fruit, biscuits, sweets and drinking water.

Game parks
- Do observe the Park rules: they really are made to protect you.

2.3 First aid in the home
CUTS AND GRAZES

- Clean the wound with antiseptic and cover with a sterile (or at least clean) dressing.
- For grazes 'vaseline gauze' (fine gauze impregnated with vaseline) will prevent the dressing from sticking to the wound.
- Elastoplast of the sort that can 'breathe' (that is, not waterproof) is fine to cover small cuts, while Micropore tape, made from paper, is useful to hold a larger dressing in place, as it allows air in and does not cause allergic reactions as some fabric-based plasters do. Healing takes place best if a graze can be left open to the air, so long as it is kept clean.
- Antibiotic powder, such as Cicatrin, will help to prevent or treat infection if the wound is dirty or looks infected.
- For deep or dirty wounds a Tetanus 'booster' injection may be necessary if more than 5 years have elapsed since your last booster. If you have never had one, you should have a 3-injection course of Tetanus Toxoid vaccination (see also *Tetanus*, section 5.1).
- Sometimes, if there is serious risk of a bacterial infection from a dirty wound, a Penicillin injection or other antibiotic treatment may be advisable.

BRUISES AND SPRAINS

- Apply a cold water, ice or witch-hazel compress for 30–60 minutes, followed by a firmly supporting bandage.
- Consult a doctor as soon as possible if you think there may be a fracture, indicated by sharp severe pain on movement or weight-bearing (see also *Fractures*, section 2.4).

SCALDS AND BURNS

- If a person's clothing catches fire, wrap immediately in a heavy material, such as a rug or a blanket, to 'choke' the flames. A scald or small surface burn should immediately be plunged into cold water for at least 10 minutes.

Check to see if any of the following are present.
Reddened skin only: if necessary, apply soothing antiseptic cream but it is best not to put on anything at all.

Blistered skin: avoid breaking any blisters, and keep open and clean, or cover with sterile dry dressing or Vaseline gauze.

Charred or severely blistered skin over a wide area: seek urgent medical help. While travelling to a hospital or waiting for a doctor, keep clean by placing the person inside a thin, clean sheet or mosquito net, keeping this carefully away from the burnt areas. Control pain by giving aspirin or paracetamol: 2 tablets every 4 hours, if available, and give frequent sips of water (every 10–15 minutes) during transportation, to replace the fluid that is being lost through the burnt surface.

POISON

A poison is any substance that will temporarily or permanently damage the body when swallowed or absorbed through the skin, eyes or lungs. Many household cleaning fluids are poisons; so are most medicines and tablets if taken in larger quantities than directed on the bottle or by the doctor. Some insecticides and pesticides are poisonous if breathed in, or can be absorbed if they come into contact with the skin surface.

If someone has swallowed a poison

● Find out what type of poison has been swallowed, and take the bottle or container with you to hospital if possible.

● Give a glass of milk to drink if possible which will help to dilute, and perhaps neutralize, the poison. Water will do if there is no milk, but give several glasses if possible. (Some poisons react with small volumes of water.)

● **Never** try to make the person vomit: this can make matters worse if the vomit is inhaled inadvertently into the lungs, or if the poison burns or corrodes.

● Take the patient to hospital, carrying some milk and water with you for the journey if this is more than 20–30 minutes long. (See section 3.2.)

If someone has been in skin contact with poison

● See warning on container and follow any instructions.

● Wash the skin with large amounts of cold water, and remove any contaminated clothing.

● Take to a hospital at once if any signs of illness develop, such as dizziness, faintness, very fast heart rate or any unusual behaviour.

If someone has been poisoned by carbon monoxide

This gas is produced in car exhausts and from gas and coal-burning fires or heaters. It becomes dangerous if inhaled in concentrated form, such as in an unventilated room.

It combines with the blood so that its capacity for carrying oxygen is severely reduced.

Signs of the poisoning include headache, faintness and giddiness; vomiting; bright red lips and skin; confusion, apparent 'drunkenness'; collapse and loss of consciousness.

If you suspect carbon monoxide poisoning
- Remove the person from the source of the gas.
- Open all windows and doors to let in fresh air.
- Give artificial respiration if necessary.
- If person is conscious and not vomiting, give sips of strong, sweet coffee to drink.
- Let person rest quietly, and if oxygen is available, give this by mask for one hour.
- Take to hospital.

If someone has been poisoned by carbon tetrachloride liquid or vapour

Carbon tetrachloride is a solvent used in dry-cleaning. If drunk or inhaled it is dangerous to the liver, heart and kidneys.

Signs of poisoning include headache, hiccups; nausea, vomiting and abdominal pains; diarrhoea; drowsiness and confusion.

If you suspect carbon tetrachloride poisoning
- Remove the person from the source of the vapour.
- Give artificial respiration if necessary.
- Give oxygen by mask if available.
- If conscious and not vomiting, give milk or large amounts of water to drink.
- Take to hospital.

If someone has got a poison in the eye

- Wash the eye thoroughly with large amounts of water. Do this by holding the eye under a gentle stream of water or filling an egg-cup with water, putting the eye into the rim of the egg-cup, and lifting the head, until the egg-cup is turned upside-down over the eye. Instruct the person to open the eye, allowing the water to bathe it. Repeat several times.
- If the eye is watering, red or painful take the person to hospital after covering the eye with an eye-pad made out of clean material.

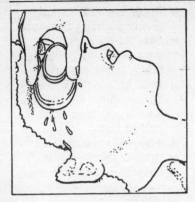

FOREIGN BODY IN THE EYE

- Try washing it out with water.
- Particles caught under the upper lid may be removed by gently turning the lid inside out and wiping the surface with a clean handkerchief or tissue.
- If the object has become embedded in the surface of the eye, do **not** attempt to remove it. Stop it damaging the eye further by covering the eye with a clean pad, and tell the person to keep both eyes shut as far as possible to minimize eye movements.

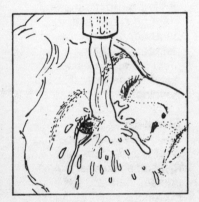

- Take the person to a hospital as soon as possible.
- Give him aspirin or paracetamol (2 tablets every 4 hours) if there is much pain.

BITES AND STINGS

It is well worth buying a book on insects or snakes if available in the country where you live. This can help in identifying the cause of a sting or bite quickly.

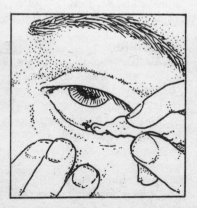

BEES
- Sterilize a needle by holding in a flame for a few seconds. Gently remove the sting, being careful not to squeeze out more poison.

- Soothe the area with antihistamine cream such as Anthisan, or apply bicarbonate of soda mixed with a small amount of water. (Do not use Anthisan in bright sunlight.)
- Occasionally severe allergic reactions occur such as rashes, or swelling of the face. If this occurs, give Piriton 4mg, and if this does not help within ½ – ¾ hour, or the person quickly becomes worse, go to a hospital as soon as possible.

WASPS
- Apply dilute vinegar.
- For allergic rashes give Piriton as above.

SCORPIONS

Most scorpions are not dangerous to adults (although their stings are still very painful), but medical help should be sought if a young child is stung. Avoid their stings by not walking bare-foot, indoors or out, but 'knock out' shoes before putting them on, and always look before you touch!

Treatment
- If a doctor is available, local anaesthetic can be injected at the site of the sting.

- Apply ice, TCP, Dettol or similar soothing antiseptic.
- Take 2 aspirin or paracetamol at once and repeat every 4 hours.
- Treat for shock by loosening tight clothing, keeping warm but not hot, lying down if pale or faint.
- If a small child develops signs of shock, a journey to hospital may be necessary.

SPIDERS

Spider bites can be painful but are seldom dangerous. Treat for shock and, if necessary, give 2 aspirin or paracetamol for pain. Small children do sometimes need hospital treatment if shock develops.

SNAKES

Bites are not common and death is very rare as a result of snakebite. But, of course, there are some poisonous snakes in most countries of the world, and they are particularly common in hot countries.

Prevention
- Always wear shoes (boots in known snake country, checking them before putting on!) and do not walk where you cannot see, especially at night.

Signs of shock are: paleness, sweating, vomiting, severe weakness or faintness, and a thready, thin pulse (difficult to feel).

- Use a torch when going into dark huts, chicken pens, stores and so on.
- Do not feel on ledges where you cannot see: **always look before you touch**!

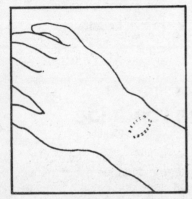

A bite from a non-poisonous snake.

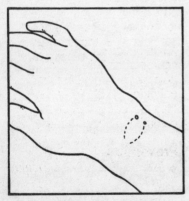

A bite from a poisonous snake.

What you should do if you are bitten

- If possible, the snake should be killed and identified. **Do not touch it** but pick it up with a cleft stick and take it with you to the hospital.
- Look for teeth marks at the site of the wound. If the snake was poisonous, 2 deep fang-marks (puncture wounds) will show. If non-poisonous, rows of smaller teeth marks will be seen, without any puncture marks.
- If non-poisonous, treat for pain with aspirin or paracetamol, and re-assure.
- If poisonous, or you are unsure, move the bitten part as little as possible and keep it lower than the heart.
- Remove any venom lying on the skin and wash the bite with lots of whatever liquid is available. Apply ice if possible.
- Tie a firm bandage along the whole length of the arm or leg to slow down the circulation but not to stop it.
- **Go to a hospital** so that anti-venin can be given, within 3 hours if possible.
- See section 3.2 for how you can help on the journey to hospital.
- Give 2 aspirin or paracetamol for pain, but **not** alcohol.
- If the **eyes** have been hit by the venom of a spitting cobra, wash out with large amounts of water, and go to a hospital as quickly as possible.

DOGS AND OTHER ANIMALS

Beware of rabies

Suspect any unprovoked attack. If the animal is alive 10 days after the bite it cannot have been rabid when it bit you.

What to do if you are bitten

The rabies virus is carried in the animal's saliva. Therefore

- Wash out the bite with large amounts of soap and water, then 70% alcohol.
- Note state of dog if it is still around, and isolate it so that it can be observed for 10 days.
- **Go to a hospital.**
For further information, see *Rabies*, section 5.1.

2.4 First aid at the roadside

(For children see special note)

IF THE INJURED PERSON IS NOT BREATHING

Carry out mouth-to-mouth artificial respiration and cardiac massage as follows:

1 Immediately place the casualty on a firm surface. Loosen his or her clothing and clear the mouth and throat of blood clot, loose teeth or any other obstruction.

2 If there is no pulse or heartbeat, stimulate the heart by placing the heel of your hand on the middle section of the person's breastbone, cover it with the heel of the other hand and press downwards sharply. Press down and release at about one 'beat' per second 5 times.

3 Tilt the head back to extend neck. Lift the jaw forward to keep the tongue out of the air passage and pinch nostrils to prevent air leakage. Take a deep breath and seal the casualty's lips firmly with yours. Blow through your mouth until you see the chest rise. Take your mouth away and allow the air to escape.

4 Alternate one 'breath' with 5 'heartbeats'. (Listen for snoring or gurgling, signs of obstruction which should be cleared). Continue in this way for up to 45 minutes or so if there are **any** signs of life at all. Stop after that if there are none.

5 As soon as breathing occurs spontaneously, turn the person onto one side to prevent inhalation of vomit or other obstruction to the airway.

Get the person to hospital as soon as possible.

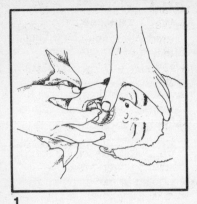

1

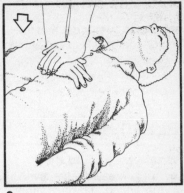

2

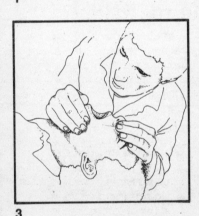

3

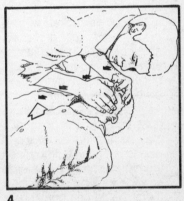

4

See further under section 3.2 for ways to help on a journey to hospital. Mouth-to-mouth artificial respiration and cardiac massage can be done during the journey.

Special note: Children

Apply light pressure to the rib cage, using fingertips only, and expand the lungs by means of small puffs, at a faster rate than for adults. Seal both nose and mouth with your lips.

DROWNING

What you should do

If the drowned person is not breathing, follow the instructions for mouth-to-mouth artificial respiration and cardiac massage.

As only small amounts of water can enter the lungs, there is no need to waste time trying to remove it. Turn a child upside-down to drain away what water there is, but do not spend more than 15 seconds at the most on this. **Every minute is precious**, and the important thing is to get air into the lungs and to get the blood circulation going again as quickly as possible.

BLEEDING

What you should do

● Apply pressure directly to the wound and bandage a clean dressing tightly against it.

● If it becomes soaked with blood, add further dressings and increase the pressure.

● Elevate the wounded part, but splint broken or dislocated bones first.

● As a last resort, if bleeding does not stop, a tourniquet may be applied above the wound if it is on a limb. The tourniquet should be at least as wide as a hand and there should be unbroken skin between it and the wound edge. It should be tightened enough to stop bleeding, but must be released for 1 minute in every 10 minutes, or permanent damage may be caused.

● Take the injured person to a hospital.

It is a good idea to carry a note of your blood group when travelling.

FRACTURES

Suspect a fracture if there is severe sharp pain, tenderness and inability to move the injured part. There may be signs of shock: paleness, sweating, vomiting, severe weakness or faintness, and a thready, thin pulse (difficult to feel).

Fractured ribs will be sharply painful on deep breathing or coughing or movements involving the chest, and there will be marked tenderness on pressure at the site of the pain. A fractured spine will be severely painful at the site of the injury or there may be pain down the legs or loss of sensation and inability to move them.

What you should do

● Move the casualty as little as possible.

● Do **not** try to move injured joints or to push exposed bone ends back into place. Cover the wounds with a clean dressing.

● Immobilize the fracture by the use of splints or a sling. (A fractured leg may be bound to its opposite number and bony areas, such as between knees and ankles, should be padded. An arm may be bound to the body with a broad strip of material.) Dislocated joints should be immobilized in the same way.

● If you suspect a spinal fracture, **move person only with extreme care**. Roll onto a stretcher or board which acts as a splint, and wrap a cover round both to prevent movement.

● Take the injured person to a hospital as soon as possible. See further in section 3.2 for ways to help on a journey to hospital.

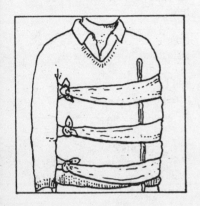

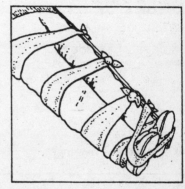

3 CHECK LIST

3.1 When to travel to hospital or call a doctor

ACUTE OR SUDDEN ONSET OF ILLNESS

In case of accident

If the answer to any of the questions below is yes, take the patient to a hospital or doctor as quickly as possible.

- Is there any difficulty with breathing?
- Is there any external bleeding which cannot easily be controlled by direct pressure? Bleeding in spurts may mean a cut artery; bleeding from ears may mean a skull fracture; bleeding from nose is not usually serious unless it continues for more than half an hour.
- Is there a rapid, thready pulse which is difficult to feel; increasing pallor and sweating? These are signs of shock and may indicate internal bleeding. If the patient is unconscious there may also be a continuing or deepening coma. If conscious there may be increasing faintness or drowsiness as well as signs of shock.
- Are there any signs of a fracture? An arm or leg will be sharply painful on movement with increasing swelling and bruising.
- Have you been attacked by a dog or animal without provocation? Do you think it may be rabid?
- Have you been bitten by a snake you think may be poisonous?
  (See also section 2.2 for accidents at home and on the road.)

In case of sudden illness

If the answer to any of the questions below is yes take the patient to a hospital or doctor as quickly as possible.

- Is there any difficulty with breathing?
- Is pain or the general condition of the patient becoming worse within a matter of 3–4 hours?
- Has vomiting occurred half-hourly or more frequently for 3 hours, or has vomiting (not just retching) occurred more than 6 times in 12 hours?
- In cases of diarrhoea, is it accompanied by fever and severe abdominal pain even between attacks?

- Is fresh red blood being passed with diarrhoea? This indicates bleeding from low down in the gut. A small amount of blood mixed with the stool is not serious unless it persists for more than one week.
- Are stools black and tarry with increasing signs of general weakness? This may mean bleeding from high up in the gut.
- Are the tongue and mouth dry, the eyes sunken, and does the skin not flatten out at once when pinched up (loss of elasticity)? Is there increasing drowsiness, and little thirst? In babies, is the fontanelle sunken? All these are signs that the person is 'drying out' (dehydration).
- Has the temperature remained above 38.5°C/101°F, even with aspirin or paracetamol 4-hourly and tepid sponging, for more than 24 hours?
- Does the temperature repeatedly rise to more than 39.5°C/103°F preceded by severe shivering attacks?

GRADUAL ONSET OF CHRONIC ILLNESSES

If the answer to any of the following questions is yes, arrange to see a doctor as soon as convenient.

- Is there weight loss of more than 7lb/3–4kg in an adult, in spite of not deliberately dieting over a period of 2–3 months or less? In small children who should be growing, any weight loss that is not quickly regained should be investigated.
- Is there persistent or recurrent pain, diarrhoea, nausea and vomiting, or high temperature?
- Is there persistent or recurrent depression, anxiety, tension, insomnia, or tiredness?
- Are there any symptoms that are increasing in severity?
- Is the problem interfering with your efficiency and effectiveness at work, or with your relationships?
- Have you found a lump or swelling you have not noticed before? See a doctor as soon as possible. If the lump or swelling has been present earlier, such as a mole, is it changing, becoming bigger or bleeding?
- Is there any unexpected blood loss in any form?
- Are there any persistent or recurrent changes in the pattern of your bowel movements or in passing urine?
- Are there any other problems you feel may be caused by illness?

3.2 What to do on a journey to hospital
OR WHILE WAITING FOR MEDICAL HELP

- Company helps, but remember, someone who is ill does not necessarily feel like chatting or even listening to someone talking to them. Just *be* with them, hold their hand, wipe away sweat, cool with a wet flannel — and be sensitive to their likely needs and wants. Do not fuss!

- Ensure a steady supply of drinks, just a few sips at a time, at 10-minute intervals or so. Someone who is vomiting or has diarrhoea needs this even more. Insist they keep sipping small quantities of fluids to replace what they are losing. The stomach will reject large quantities taken all at once, but should retain fluid that is 'dripped' in. For small children and babies this is **essential**: they become dehydrated more quickly than adults. If necessary, feed the fluid to them continuously by teaspoon.

- Ensure there is nothing blocking or hindering breathing.

- If the patient has a pain or a temperature, 4-hourly aspirin or paracetamol will help to some extent.

- Someone who has a high temperature will need to have a good through-draught of air to help cool them down; sponge them down with tepid or cool water from time to time, and do not cover them with a lot of clothing, which will only cause them to retain the heat. Shivering usually means a temperature is rising in someone who is ill and feverish.

- Someone with a (suspected) fracture must have the limb immobilized in some way for the journey. Strap one injured leg to the other, or strap an arm to the body, or use a splint. (See also *Fractures*, section 2.4.)

- Someone who is ill is often frightened. This might make them appear over-anxious and aggressive. Respond calmly, keep your own fears to yourself, but accept the person's anxiety. It does not help to be told not to be silly or to stop worrying. Reassurances like, 'Yes, I know it hurts; I know it's worrying, but we'll get you to hospital as soon as possible, and meanwhile I'll stay right here with you' are more helpful.

● If the patient is unconscious: place in the recovery position (see *First aid*, section 2.4) and prop up with pillows to keep the patient well-anchored in that position; ensure the airway is clear; and stay with the patient to keep constant check on these things. See also under *First aid* for advice about bleeding from an injury or other problems.

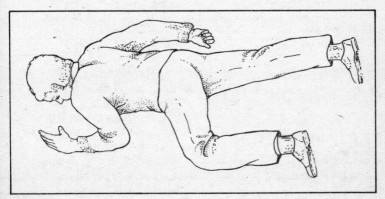

The recovery position.

4 TRAVELLING

Here is a check list of things that have to do with general health to help you if you are planning to travel abroad. There is also a suggested timetable for immunizations. A suggested first-aid kit is to be found in section 2.1.

4.1 Check List

PLANNING YOUR JOURNEY

Try to think at least 3 months ahead.

- Plan your Immunizations. Check the list later in this section to see which are necessary, and see the suggested timetable for planning them.
- Have a dental check-up and any necessary treatment. Nothing is more miserable than a toothache to spoil your travels! Make sure you have a spare set of dentures if you need them.
- Have your eyes checked. Do you need new glasses or sunglasses? Make sure you take a spare set with you. If you use contact lenses, take a spare set, or a pair of spare glasses, and ensure you have a supply of the cleaning solution with you.

- Ensure you have a 1–3 month supply of your usual contraceptive Pill or other medication with you, and that you know whether or not you can get more in the area to which you are going. If you cannot, make sure you have a 'supply-line' organized.
- Ensure you have found out if you require anti-malarial tablets. Start taking them 1–2 weeks before you go to give you adequate protection and to ensure they do not cause you any side-effects. See the section on malaria for more advice. Remember you may be bitten by the mosquito that carries malaria if your plane stops at an airport in a malarious area.
- Make up your own first-aid kit. See section 2.1 for suggestions.
- Take out insurance to cover accidental injury, illness and dental treatment in the country to which you are going, or while travelling. Ensure you know what it covers and how to set about getting emergency help and finances should you require them.
- IAMAT (International Association for Medical Assistance to Travellers) provides a useful service. It

has a list of good doctors available to travellers in a large number of countries, information about climate and the risks of such illnesses as malaria and schistosomiasis.

IMMUNIZATIONS

Explanatory notes

These notes are intended to be used in conjunction with the Plan of action: Timetable and Check list.

Different parts of the world have different disease patterns. You will need to check with your doctor, travel agent, vaccination centre or local department of health to find out which vaccinations are essential or recommended for the various parts of the world.

The commonly recommended ones are listed here. They have been dealt with in the same order in which they appear in the check list. You will notice that certain vaccines have been marked as being 'live': this means that the organism used in the vaccine is still alive, although it has been 'treated' in such a way as to weaken (attenuate) it. It will not cause illness in this form but will still provoke the immune response of the body's defence mechanism. The importance of this, here, is that

you will need to remember, as you plan your immunization schedule, that live vaccinations should *either* be given at the same time *or* with an interval of *3 weeks*. The others can be given at the same time as each other or with the live ones.

At any time before the last two months

Find out if you need to have any of the following, and if you do, arrange to start your courses as soon as possible.

● **BCG against tuberculosis**
BCG is a live vaccine. If you have had a BCG in the past then you will be immune already, and need do nothing further. Some will have had skin tests (called Heaf or Mantoux tests) done at school to check if they are immune. If the test was positive, then again you need do nothing further. However, if you do not know whether or not you are immune, ask your doctor to arrange for you to have a skin test. If it is negative you will need to have a BCG vaccination done if you are going to a country where there is a lot of TB. It is not necessary if you are only going for a holiday or short stay.

The BCG vaccination will raise a small nodule in the skin which will last for several weeks, and may also cause a small ulcer. There may be swollen glands under the arm; all these will gradually settle down and leave only a small scar on the skin at the site of the vaccination.

BCG vaccination gives life-long immunity, and is advised also for babies and small children. It can be given immediately after birth. (See also *Tuberculosis*, section 6.)

● TETANUS TOXOID against 'lock-jaw' or tetanus

Many will have had a full course (often as part of the Triple vaccination) when they were babies, with a pre-school booster, and, perhaps, another booster dose when they have cut themselves. If you are one of these people then one booster dose will be sufficient if it is less than 10 years since your last one.

If it is more than 10 years since your last booster then you will need to have a full course of 3 injections: 2 with an interval of 1 month, followed by a third 6 months or so later.

If you have never had a course then you should have the full course of 3 injections. Keep up the boosters every 5–10 years.

● YELLOW FEVER

Yellow fever is a live vaccine. It is a very effective vaccination which will give protection for 10 years. You will have to go to a special yellow fever vaccination centre, which will issue an international certificate. This vaccination could be done as soon as you know you are going to, or through, a country which requires it. If time is very short it can be given in the last couple of weeks, together with the gamma-globulin (which does not reduce the immune response to the yellow fever vaccination).

● RUBELLA — against German Measles

Rubella is a live vaccine. This vaccination is for women of child-bearing age, or any girl of 10 years and over. (In some countries it is given to girls at 15 months). It is very effective and will give life-long immunity. A blood test can be done to check if you are already immune. If you are not, arrange to have one, but remember the following:
● Be absolutely certain you are not pregnant.
● Avoid pregnancy for 3 months after the vaccination.

- Avoid any pregnant women for 3 weeks afterwards, in case you infect them.
- You should not have a yellow fever or BCG vaccination within 3 weeks of the injection: there should be 3 weeks between any 'live' vaccinations. Note also that there should be 6 weeks between having a skin test for TB (see above under *BCG*) and the rubella vaccine. (See also *German measles*, section 5.4.)

● HEPATITIS B vaccine

This is an effective vaccine against the type of hepatitis that is passed on by blood-to-blood contact. It is usually available only to those who are at particular risk (doctors, dentists, nurses or midwives). If you are likely to be at risk through your work, arrange with your doctor to have the course of 3 injections: the vaccine has to be specially ordered for you. There should be an interval of 1 month between the first 2 injections, then 6 months till the third.

● POLIO vaccine

Polio is a live oral vaccine. Poliomyelitis is still very widespread in most developing countries and it is important to ensure protection against it. Many people have a full course when they are babies, with a booster given just before going to school.

For those who have not had a course, or for whom it is more than 10 years since the last booster dose, start a full course of 3 oral doses with 1 month interval between each. If it is less than 10 years, you should have 1 booster dose before you go.

In the final two months

● RABIES

There is now a very effective vaccine against rabies known as the Human Diploid Cell Vaccine. A full course consists of 3 injections, the first 2 separated by an interval of 1 month, the third, as a booster or reinforcement, 6–12 months later. However, the first 2 injections will give some protection for about 2 years, so if you do not have time to fit in the full course it is sufficient to have just the 2.

Whether you have 2 or 3 injections, always keep in

NOTE
'Live' vaccines should either be given at the same time as another 'live' one, or with a 3 week interval.

mind that you **must go to a hospital immediately** if you are bitten by a suspect dog (*any* unprovoked attack by a dog, or other mammal, is suspect — see *Rabies*, section 5.1 for further information).

Those at special risk through their work (agricultural workers and vets, for example) may be entitled to the immunization free though it has to be ordered specially for you by your doctor. Others have to go to a vaccination centre or order it directly from the manufacturers through their doctor. It is expensive, but worth having if you are going to live in a country where rabies is common.

● **TYPHOID**
The vaccine used against this disease is about 70% effective, but is definitely worth having as some protection is very much better than none against what can be a serious illness.

The usual course is 2 injections with an interval of between 10 days to 8 weeks. This will give you adequate protection for 3 years (except in some areas with very high incidence of typhoid). One injection will give immunity for 1 year, so if you are only going to be at risk for a short time, or

time for preparation is short, then 1 dose is sufficient. A booster after 1 year is then advisable if you prolong your stay.

● **CHOLERA**
The vaccine used against this disease is not very effective and for this reason very few countries now require an international certificate of vaccination against it. One injection is sufficient to satisfy any requirements and will also give some immunity for about 6 months. The full course is 2 doses separated by between 10 days to 4 weeks, but does not give appreciably better immunity, nor does it last any longer.

In the last two weeks

● **GAMMA-GLOBULIN**
If you know you have had hepatitis A (infectious hepatitis) then you do not need to have this protection as you will already have an immunity.

For those who have not had this illness, the passive protection provided by gamma-globulin, although not 100%, is definitely worth having. The protection lasts only 4 – 6 months, but as the illness can leave you weak and depressed for several months, it is of value, especially if you are only going for a short stay. In some countries, where hepatitis A is very common, it is advisable to have gamma-globulin every 6 months if it is available. It can also be of value to have an injection of gamma-globulin if you know you have had contact with hepatitis A or if there is an epidemic.

You should have the injection in the last week or so before you go in order to give you maximum protection on arrival.

NOTE

There is now a theoretical risk of the AIDS virus being transmitted through gamma-globulin as it is made from blood-products but the manufacturing process should kill the virus.

● SMALLPOX

This is no longer required or necessary as the illness has been eradicated thanks to the work of the World Health Organization and health workers co-operating throughout the world.

● OTHERS

There are vaccinations against mumps, meningitis and Japanese B encephalitis which may also be recommended for specific areas.

PLAN OF ACTION: TIMETABLE AND CHECK LIST

THINK 3 MONTHS AHEAD — OR MORE!

As soon as you know that you are going abroad, check through the following timetable, and together with the explanatory notes work out your own schedule of immunizations and check it off as you deal with each item. If you do not have 3 months or more, see the explanatory notes for advice.

AT ANY TIME BEFORE THE LAST 2 MONTHS	DURING THE LAST 2 MONTHS	IN THE LAST 2 WEEKS
*BCG — skin test first — single dose, if required	*RABIES — 2 doses — can be given to children over 6 months old	GAMMA-GLOBULIN — single dose

AT ANY TIME BEFORE THE LAST 2 MONTHS	DURING THE LAST 2 MONTHS	IN THE LAST 2 WEEKS
TETANUS — booster or a full course of 3 injections	months old TYPHOID — 2 doses	Start anti-malarials
*YELLOW FEVER — single dose if required — can be given to children over 9 months old	CHOLERA — 2 doses These may be given at the same time	
*RUBELLA — women of child-bearing age or girls 11 years+ — single dose		
HEPATITIS B — for those at risk, a course of 3 injections (doctors, nurses, dentists)		
*POLIO — one booster or a full course		
*live vaccines and should not be given too close, if possible. If unavoidable, give on same day.		

FOR CHILDREN

Below 1 year — BCG, at birth if possible
— Triple vaccine and polio
At 1 year — Measles
Above 1 year — As for adults, plus pre-school boosters of Triple vaccine and polio

IF YOU HAVE ONLY 4–6 WEEKS PREPARATION TIME

4–6 WEEKS TO DEPARTURE

TETANUS	Booster	If no previous course, or more than 10 years since last booster, start course now with first injection.
POLIO	Booster	If no previous course, or more than 10 years since last booster, start course now with first dose.
RABIES	First injection	(if necessary for your work or going to high risk area)

2–4 WEEKS TO DEPARTURE

TYPHOID	Single dose	(or first of two if necessary; see explanatory notes)
CHOLERA	Single dose	

0–2 WEEKS TO DEPARTURE

TETANUS	Second dose	(if necessary)
RABIES	Second dose	
TYPHOID	Second dose	(if necessary)
YELLOW FEVER	Single dose	⎤
POLIO	Booster (or second dose)	⎦ > on same day
GAMMA-GLOBULIN		With the above, or just a day or two before departure if possible.

NOTES:
1. You will probably have some fever and a sore arm for a day or two.
2. You should have a third re-inforcing dose of polio after 1 month.
3. You should have a third dose of tetanus after 6 months.
4. See explanatory notes about rabies.

IF YOU HAVE NO TIME TO PREPARE

YELLOW FEVER	On the	
POLIO	same day	
TYPHOID	Single dose	
CHOLERA	Single dose	(only if absolutely necessary)
TETANUS	Booster	(if necessary)
GAMMA-GLOBULIN	Single dose	

All the above can be given on the same day, if necessary, but remember that you will have a sore arm (or site of injection!) and possibly run a fever for a day or two as you travel. The immune response of the body may not be so effective as it would have been had the injections been properly spaced.

TABLE OF COMMON IMMUNIZATIONS AND THEIR EFFECTS

Vaccine	Yellow fever	Rubella	BCG
Type	Live	Live	Live
Number of doses	1 injection	1 injection	1 injection
Boosters	10 years	if blood test is negative	if skin test is negative
Effectiveness	★★★	★★	★★
Complications	Should not be given to pregnant women or babies under 1 year	Should not be given to pregnant women; avoid pregnancy for 3 months after injections	Causes swelling or small ulcer for 6 weeks or more

NOTE
Live vaccines should not be given at the same time, and they should not be given to pregnant women.

TABLE OF COMMON IMMUNIZATIONS AND THEIR EFFECTS

Vaccine	**Typhoid**	**Polio**	**Cholera**
Type	Killed	Live oral	Killed
Number of doses	2 injections	3 doses by mouth	2 injections
			6 months
Boosters	1 – 2 years	5 years	
Effectiveness	★★	★★★	★
Complications	Painful arm, with or without fever	None usually	Painful arm, with or without fever for 1 – 2 days

Vaccine	**Tetanus**	**Gamma globulin**	**Rabies**
Type	Toxoid	Passive	Killed
Number of doses	3 injections	1 injection	2 injections initially (booster at 6 – 24 months)
Boosters	5 – 10 years	4 – 6 months	1 – 2 years
Effectiveness	★★★	★★	★★
Complications	Painful arm, with or without fever for 1 – 2 days	Only effective against 1 form of hepatitis	Post-exposure treatment still required

TABLE OF COMMON IMMUNIZATIONS AND THEIR EFFECTS

Vaccine	Diphtheria	Pertussis	Measles
Type	Toxoid	Killed	Live
Number of doses	3 injections within 1st year of life	3 injections within 1st year of life	1 injection
Boosters	Pre-school	Pre-school	
Effectiveness	★★★	★★	★★
Complications	None	Avoid if history of fits	10 days later mild fever and rash; care if egg allergy known

MALARIA

(See also section 6 for full discussion of the whole subject.)

Malaria is an increasing problem worldwide and the advice you will be given depends on the area to which you go. Even within a particular country there will be wide variations in the prevalence of the disease and in the advice given.

A person becomes infected by being bitten by an infected Anopheles mosquito. There are 4 different types of malaria bug. Only 1 of these may cause death if untreated, but the others can cause severe and recurring illness. One type can live in the body for a long time and then cause malaria many months after the person has left the area.

Prevention

1 Avoid contact with the mosquito.

- Use mosquito nets, slow burning coil or electrical repellant device.
- Avoid breeding sites, which are likely to be shaded, slightly moving, clean water; note the short flight range of less than 1 mile.
- Keep yourself covered during biting periods.
- Learn the local biting cycle, of which there are 2 main types:

a) Twilight for 1½–2 hours, stop overnight, and bite again at dawn.

b) 8.30 p.m. until 3.30 a.m., with none at dusk or dawn (malaria mosquitos never bite during the day).

● Screening the house is expensive and unreliable, but may help in heavily infested areas.

● Mosquito repellants help, but need frequent re-application.

● Lights can cut the number of bites by 50%.

2 Take regular anti-malarial drugs according to the recommendations for your area. The drugs most commonly used are the following:

● **Paludrine** (Proguanil): 100mg × 2 tablets daily.

NOTE

This is a safe drug, but will not give 100% protection.

● **Cloroquine** 150mg × 2 tablets weekly. (Dose should equal 300mg base: see *Special note*.)

NOTE

It has been customary to recommend that Cloroquine is kept to treat an attack of malaria, but its use to prevent malaria is now accepted, where there is not resistance to it. It should not be taken for more than 3 years continuously, but is a very safe drug, even in pregnancy.

● **Maloprim** 1 tablet weekly (no more!)

NOTE

This is used where there is Cloroquine resistance. Resistance to Maloprim also exists. It can cause jaundice in babies under 8 weeks, but malaria itself could be a more serious problem and so it may be necessary to give it in special circumstances. See later note also about pregnancy.

● **Daraprim** (Pyrimethamine): 1 tablet weekly.

NOTE

This is still used in some countries but resistance to it has developed in many parts of the world. However, it is useful for children as it is available as a tasteless liquid and can be given before the baby is 8 weeks old.

● **Fansidar** 1 tablet weekly.

NOTE

This should only be used where there is resistance to the other drugs. It is most useful for treating an attack of malaria and should be kept for that where possible. Resistance to this is also developing. It should not be given to pregnant women or babies under 8 weeks.

SPECIAL NOTES

1 Some of these drugs can be used in combination, Maloprim and Paludrine, for example, or Cloroquine and Paludrine. You will need to take the advice of local doctors when you arrive.

2 For those who cannot take Maloprim or Fansidar (Sulphonamide sensitivity, tendency to methaemoglobinaemia and certain blood disorders) Paludrine will give some protection and lessen the severity of the illness, so is worth taking.

3 What is the Cloroquine base?
This is the amount of actual Cloroquine available in a tablet of Cloroquine salt, such as sulphate or phosphate. It is the base amount that matters, and a note about it can be found (usually in small print) somewhere on the bottle. Nivaquine (sulphate) and Avloclor (phosphate) tablets both contain 150mg base.

You will need to check with your doctor or travel adviser which anti-malarials you should take in the areas to which you are travelling. The situation is changing so rapidly that it is impossible to give definitive advice about the exact tablets or combination of tablets you should be taking. This is because the malaria organisms are very quickly developing resistance to many anti-malarials. New anti-malarial drugs are constantly being researched all over the world. Malaria vaccine is a possibility for the future, but as yet not available.

Start your anti-malarial medication 1–2 weeks before you start your journey, continue taking it regularly throughout your stay and for 4–6 weeks after leaving the malarious area. See a doctor if any fever occurs after a stay in a malarious area.

Treatment of an attack

● Take 4 tablets of Cloroquine (150mg base × 4) immediately.

● Take 2 tablets of Cloroquine (150mg base × 2) 6 hours later.

● Take 2 tablets of Cloroquine (150mg base × 2) on the mornings of the second, third and fourth days.
OR

● Take Fansidar, 2 tablets at once if weight is under 63.5kg/10st, otherwise 3 tablets. Repeat if necessary 7 days later, but not sooner. Dosage for children in an attack of malaria when using Fansidar: 9–14 years, 2 tablets; 4–8 years, 1 tablet; under 4 years, ½ tablet.

For children, use the same drugs as recommended for adults except in the first 8 weeks of life, when Cloroquine or Paludrine are best if possible. Children of all ages, including breast-fed infants, require protection. Weight is a better guide than age when estimating the dose. See dosage chart.

Pregnancy and malaria

An attack of malaria in pregnancy is dangerous both to mother and baby, so preventive treatment is essential. Cloroquine and Paludrine are safe to take during pregnancy, but Maloprim and Fansidar are not recommended by the manufacturers. Although there are no proven cases of foetal malformation with either in the doses used to prevent the disease, there is a small risk. This small risk must be weighed against the much greater risk of an actual attack of malaria in an area where there is a high level of Cloroquine resistance.

This is a difficult problem with no easy answer. If it is possible to delay going abroad to a resistant area until after the birth of the baby, then this would be preferable. Likewise, if it is possible to delay starting a family until after returning to a non-resistant or non-malarious area, this again would be best. However, if these options are not open to you, remember that no pregnancy anywhere can be guaranteed risk-free, and the risks of malaria in pregnancy are enormous compared to those of taking the anti-malarial during pregnancy. The risks of taking Maloprim can be minimized by taking folic acid 5mg daily if there is any likelihood of your being pregnant.

4.2 Health hints while travelling

FLYING

Jet lag

Remember the biological clock. When flying from east to west or vice versa, you may cross time zones, gaining or losing several hours. Your 'body clock' will take some days to become synchronized to the local time, and you should spend at least the first day after the air journey resting quietly if possible.

Dehydration

Drink plenty of non-alcoholic fluids. The dry air in the

aeroplane will dry you out a great deal. Much of the tiredness from air travel results from not drinking enough. Both you and your children should have a constant supply of water or soft drinks. If you are not offered them, get up and get them yourself or ask for them. Alcoholic drinks (often offered free and therefore a great temptation) are dehydrating, so be strict about limiting the amount of alcohol you drink.

Motion sickness or travel sickness

Most people are not travel sick while flying, but some people are particularly susceptible. If you have not been in an aeroplane before, take some anti-nausea tablets (such as Marzine, Sea-Legs, Stugeron, Kwells or Avomine) with you, in case you find you do become nauseated. If you know you do, take the tablets ½ – ¾ hour before departure time, but remember you will feel drowsy, and do not drink alcohol.

If you have children with you who have not flown before, do not suggest to them that they might be sick: this may frighten them and make them more likely to feel unwell. Do not keep asking them, either, if they are all right: they will tell you soon enough if they are not! However, give them the appropriate dose ½ – ¾ hour before departure time if they

have had previous experience of motion sickness, but remember they will feel drowsy and perhaps be a bit miserable. They will need to have plenty of games to play and books to read; boredom contributes to the 'miseries' as much as anything. Sometimes sucking peppermints or sweets with ginger in them will help reduce the feeling of nausea. The above comments also apply to car sickness.

Ear Troubles

Aircraft are pressurized, but not sufficiently for the pressure to remain absolutely the same at sea level as at 11,000m/36,000 feet! Some people feel their ears 'popping' as the plane takes off, or more often, when it is landing. Sucking sweets, yawning or blowing your nose will help to equalize the pressure between the atmospheric pressure in the aircraft and behind the ear drum (it is the difference that causes the discomfort).

Severe pain is sometimes felt if you are prone to catarrh or sinusitis, or happen to have a cold when travelling because the Eustachian tube between the ear and the nose becomes blocked and it is difficult to 'equalize' the pressures. If you know you have this trouble, ½ – 1 Actifed (or similar decongestant) tablet (or some Ephedrine nose drops) ½ – ¾ hour before take off or landing, may help to unblock the tubes and keep them open during the crucial pressure changes. Remember, however, that Actifed can cause drowsiness.

Other common problems

- Swollen feet will settle within hours or within a day or two of landing. Do not take your shoes off on the aircraft — you may not be able to get them on again! Do not wear tight shoes for travelling in any case, and walk up and down the aisle from time to time.
- Your stomach may feel rather bloated because any gases you have in your intestines expand at high altitudes. Do not wear tight clothing as this will increase your discomfort.
- Do not go to sleep with your legs crossed because the blood in your calf veins could get blocked and even clot if you do not move for a few hours.

People with special health problems

- If you have had a recent abdominal operation, or one involving your ears or nose, please check with your doctor that it is safe for you to travel: the expansion of gases could cause problems. (See *Ear problems*, section 5.1.)
- If you have had a recent heart attack, or have a chronic chest or blood-pressure problem, please check with your doctor that it is safe for you to travel. The oxygen supply at high altitudes is lower than at sea level, and you may not be fit to cope with a lower level of oxygen than you are used to. If you have to travel, tell the stewardess so that she can ensure that you have a supply of oxygen available.
- People who are severely anaemic, or who have sickle cell disease should also ensure a supply of oxygen is available. Do not sit in the smoking area: even if you are not smoking yourself, the smoking of other people reduces the oxygen supply even further. If you have any other specific problems, such as diabetes, discuss it with your doctor, but stick to your usual medication and times until arrival and adjust then.

Flying phobias

Some unfortunate people are really frightened by flying. If you are one of these, see your doctor to discuss taking a small supply of a tranquillizer to help you during the flight. A good one is Diazepam (2 or 5mg, the effect of which lasts 12 hours or more) or Clobazam (10mg, the effect of which lasts 6 hours or so), but remember they may make you drowsy.

4.3 Health hints while acclimatizing

General

After you leave the air part of the journey make it a rule to carry a plastic container of safe water with you, some aspirin for headaches, sunglasses for glare, a hat and sun protection lotion. If you are subject to travel sickness see previous note about what to take.

Sun and heat

● **Sunburn:** for those who have not experienced the intense heat and sun of the tropics and some other areas, remember that the effects can be quite drastic. Treat the sun with respect. If you are sunbathing, do so for 10 to 15 minutes at a time. Double this time after a few days, and gradually increase according to your needs. Use high protection (factor 5 or more) sun tan lotions, especially if you are fair skinned and have blond or red hair. Wear a sun hat and sun-glasses while you are acclimatizing.

● **Fluid loss:** sweating increases the loss of fluid and salt. It is important that you replace what you are losing through your skin by drinking much more than usual, but not alcohol, tea or coffee! These are all dehydrating and will actually make you feel worse. The colour of your urine should remain pale, indicating that it is well-diluted. The salt loss can be made up by adding some extra to your food, but do not overdo it. The sweating mechanism is inefficient initially, and it takes 1 to 2 weeks to adjust to the hotter climate. After 2 weeks you can reduce your fluid and salt intake to whatever is comfortable unless you are someone who continues to perspire very profusely.

● **Comfort and hygiene:** light, loose clothes, especially cotton, are the most comfortable to wear as they allow ventilation and cooling, and absorb some of the perspiration. Shower, or wash, splashing water over yourself from a bucket or basin, at least once or twice a day if possible.

Traveller's diarrhoea

This is very common soon after arrival in another country. It is usually mild, lasts for 24–36 hours, and treatment with antibiotics is best avoided. The danger lies in dehydration and the treatment is to replace fluid and salts lost by drinking extra safe fluids of whatever sorts are available: diluted fruit juices are particularly good. (For further information, see next section.)

Food
Try out the new foods, but remember your stomach may also need to 'acclimatize', and do not overdo the experimenting. Beware of food from street vendors, initially at least, and be especially wary of seafoods: many oceans and beaches are the local sewage disposal area!

Water
Beware of the water until you have checked it is safe. Even in prestigious hotels it can be contaminated. It is a good idea to carry a small electric coil. Put this into a mug or jug of water in a hotel room to boil it before you drink it or use it for brushing teeth. Use water sterilizing tablets as an alternative but these are not 100% effective and do leave a taste.

Allow the first minute or so of the hotel shower water to run before getting under it: this will allow bacteria to be washed away from the shower head (especially useful to prevent Legionnaire's disease).

4.4 Health hints while living abroad

WATER
Always find out that it is safe before you drink any water. Do not assume that it is safe because it comes out of a tap.

Possible sources of water
● Surface water such as rivers, dams and so on: this is likely to be very contaminated, unless there is a really effective filtration plant.
● Wells: surface wells are often very contaminated unless there is a surrounding wall and a cover, but deep tube wells usually provide clean safe water.
● Rain-water (collected from the roof): may be fairly clean, but will still need filtering.

Storage of water
All visible particles should be allowed to settle to the bottom of the container, which should be cleaned regularly. Large quantities of water should be stored in covered containers

such as earthenware jars. These are excellent, and they are also good for keeping the water cool. (Note that sedimentation takes place more quickly at room temperature than in a refrigerator.)

Purifying water for drinking

If your supply is obviously dirty, filter it first. The best filter is the ceramic type, which is effective for a long time and will filter out many disease organisms. Filter papers are quite good too. However, filtering is not as foolproof as boiling, and you should filter first, then boil (in case the filter is contaminated). Boiling is the safest way to sterilize water. You will kill all major disease organisms if you boil briskly for 5–7 minutes. Boiling for 20 minutes or so is unnecessary and could concentrate unwanted chemicals. Since water boils at a lower temperature at higher altitudes, you will have to boil it for at least 10 minutes there, and keep the lid on to conserve the steam.

SPECIAL NOTES
- Use boiled water for cleaning teeth.
- Babies often drink the bath water. Therefore, heat the water for the bath to near boiling, then allow to cool to the appropriate temperature. Otherwise, use rain-water for bathing babies, if possible, when boiling is not so necessary.
- Sterilizing tablets, containing chlorine, can be useful when travelling, but they will not work if the water is visibly dirty. Allow such water to stand first, until the dirt settles, then pour off the cleaner water. Use sterilizing tablets only if it is impossible for you to boil the water.
- Filtering does **not** get rid of viruses: they are much smaller than bacteria.

WATER-BORNE DISEASES CAUSING DIARRHOEA

These include:
- Gastro-enteritis and dysentery
- Typhoid
- Cholera

The danger in diarrhoeal illnesses lies in dehydration. This is especially true in babies and young children.

Treatment of diarrhoea

The important thing is to replace the losses of water and salt. **Drink extra fluid**. This may be all that is necessary in a mild case. Almost any fluid will do, but fruit squashes, Coca Cola and other carbonated drinks are particularly good.

REHYDRATION SOLUTION

For more severe cases, and for babies, make up this rehydration drink

Water	1 litre
Sugar	8 teaspoons
Salt	½ teaspoon
Sodium bicarbonate	¼ teaspoon (or better still sodium citrate)

Don't overdo the salt! It should taste no saltier than tears. Give 2 large cups for each loose stool in adults, one cup for babies. Even cholera can be successfully treated in this way. Dioralyte and Oralyte Packets contain the above mixture, accurately measured, and are good but expensive.

NOTES
- Continue to breast-feed a baby while giving extra fluid.
- Start treatment when the diarrhoea starts: don't wait for signs of dehydration.
- Continue to give the fluid even if there is vomiting: some of it is being absorbed, especially if given as sips only, or by teaspoon every 10–15 minutes.
- Treat throughout the night if necessary, working in shifts.
- Medication does not cure and may prolong the illness, though it soothes the symptoms. Try Diocalm, Codeine Phosphate, Imodium, Kaolin mixtures.

(For more detailed information about diarrhoea, see *First-aid kit*, section 2.1; also *Diarrhoea*, sections 5.1 and 5.4; *Common drugs*, section 8.)

NOTE
Other common water-borne diseases include
- Hepatitis A
- Polio

FOOD
See also *Nutrition*, section 1.1

Storage
Store food where it cannot be contaminated by flies, cockroaches or ants.

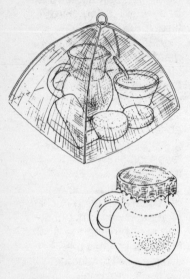

Milk
All milk should be boiled.

Yoghurt
This should be made with boiled milk. It is often helpful in treating diarrhoea.

Butter and cheese
If possible, either eat only well-known brands or make your own.

Fruit, vegetables and salads
These should be thoroughly washed in boiled or chlorinated water. Beware of salads in cafés or even some hotels: they may have been washed in contaminated water!

Cream and ice-cream
These may be contaminated and should be avoided, unless you know who has made it.

Ice-cubes
Avoid them unless you have made them yourself in case they have been made with contaminated water.

Fish and meat
Ensure this is properly cooked and do not reheat from the previous day unless well refrigerated.

Seafoods
Beware of these and eat only if properly cooked. Many beaches and shores are the local sewage disposal area!

5 SPECIFIC MEDICAL ADVICE

5.1 Adults, general: A–Z

ABDOMINAL PAIN

Causes include:

Indigestion: pain or discomfort after a heavy or spicy meal, in the upper abdomen, sometimes a burning sensation up towards the throat, with wind and nausea. See *Indigestion*.

Peptic ulcer: pain in the upper abdomen, worse before or after meals and at night, often relieved by food, milk and antacids. See *Ulcers*.

Hepatitis: right-sided upper abdominal pain, with loss of appetite, nausea, sometimes vomiting, flu-like symptoms, jaundice, dark urine and pale stools. See *Hepatitis*.

Gall stones: sudden, severe, upper right-sided pain, often after fatty meals. See *Gall Stones*.

Colic: pain that comes in waves, often leading to diarrhoea; may also cause distress in babies. See *Colic*.

Appendicitis: pain starts in upper or central abdomen, settles lower right and will be accompanied by nausea, some vomiting and low-grade fever; the lower right side becomes tender to touch or on pressure, and it becomes difficult to stand up straight. See *Appendicitis*.

Urinary problems: pain may radiate to the back and genitalia; may be accompanied by frequent passing of urine and discomfort in the lower part of the abdomen. See *Cystitis*.

Period pains: lower abdomen, sometimes back, often spasmodic. See *Menstrual problems*, section 5.3.

Constipation: may cause severe pain, especially in left side, but often general. See appropriate sections of the book for treatment of these pains. See *Constipation*.

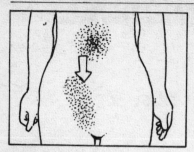

Appendicitis
Pain moves from central position to lower right. Accompanied by constipation, nausea and low fever.

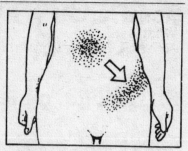

Colic and diarrhoea or dysentery
Pain is often central at first. Relieved by using the toilet.

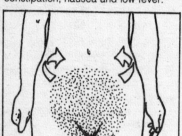

Period pain
Radiates to one side, or both, and sometimes to back and thighs.

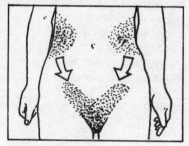

Urinary problems
Pain radiates to back and genital region. Passing water is painful and frequent and there may be high fever.

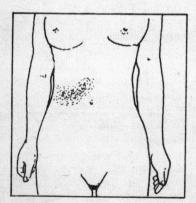

Hepatitis
Flu-like symptoms with jaundice, dark urine and pale stools.

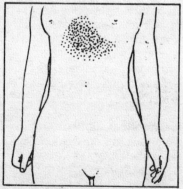

Ulcer or dyspepsia
Worse before meals and at night. Relieved by food, milk and antacids.

ACNE
What is it?

Acne is an unsightly eruption of small and large spots on the face, back and upper chest, occurring especially in teenagers, but sometimes in older people. It is associated with hormone changes.

How can it be prevented?

It cannot be completely prevented, but can be kept under control.

- Keep face, back and neck as clean as possible, using medicated soap and plenty of water.
- Avoid very fatty and sweet foods.
- Avoid squeezing black heads and white heads. If you must, then dab the spot with some alcohol (eau-de-Cologne) or TCP afterwards, having washed your hands first before touching your face.
- Eat a healthy diet with plenty of fresh fruit and vegetables.

How can it be treated?

What you can do yourself:

- Apply TCP, eau-de-Cologne or surgical spirits (after washing hands) to face and other affected areas.
- There are quite a few good preparations such as Quinoderm or Acne gel; sunlight also helps.
- Ensure you eat a good diet with plenty of fruit and vegetables, and cut down on fried foods and sweets.

If this does not help, discuss it with a doctor, who may prescribe:

- A stronger preparation to apply to the area.
- An antibiotic such as Oxytetracycline 250mg twice daily to take on a long-term basis.

Occasionally, if the problem is very severe and the above measures do not help, you may be referred to a skin specialist. Ultraviolet lamp treatment may be advised — but great care has to be taken not to burn the skin.

AIDS

See *Sexually transmitted diseases*.

ALLERGY

This is a sensitivity reaction to certain substances which are breathed in, eaten, injected or touched. Reaction can take the form of an itching rash, lumpy patches like a nettle-rash (hives), sneezing (hay fever), or itchy watering eyes. Occasionally, if the reaction is severe, there may be vomiting and diarrhoea, difficulty in breathing or shock.

Causes

Bee stings, pollen, medicines such as penicillin, foods such as shellfish or cow's milk, animal furs and insecticides are all possible causes.

How can allergies be prevented?

- If you know you are allergic to a substance, avoid it.
- Carry antihistamine tablets, such as Piriton, with you in case you are inadvertently in contact with the substance, but remember that these cause drowsiness, so do not drive or use machinery while taking them.
- If you have had an allergic reaction to a medicine, never use that medicine again; always tell any doctor or nurse who treats you in the future about the reaction.

How should allergies be treated?

What you can do yourself:

- Take an antihistamine tablet such as Piriton 4mg 3 times a day, or Phenergan 10mg twice a day, at the first signs of a reaction.
- Use Calamine Lotion to soothe itching, or Anthisan cream, but avoid using this in strong sunlight, or more than occasionally as Anthisan can cause its own allergic reaction with repeated use.
- For hay fever, take the medicine prescribed for you throughout the time you are liable to suffer symptoms.

NOTE

If you know you have a tendency to sudden and severe reactions such as sometimes occur with bee stings, an injection of Piriton 10mg may be necessary, and Piriton for injection should be carried in the first-aid kit if you are living or travelling away from medical facilities.

Anyone who does have a very severe reaction must be taken to a hospital at once. See also section 3.2 for what to do on a journey to hospital.

ANAEMIA

What is it?

It is a reduction in the oxygen-carrying part of the blood, the haemoglobin (Hb), which is the pigment contained in the red cells. Iron and some vitamins are important for its formation. Anaemia also occurs when there is a reduction in the volume and number of the cells themselves.

What causes it?

There are many causes such as:

- Blood loss: acute, as in haemorrhage from a wound or after delivery of a baby; or chronic, over a long period of time, as in women with heavy menstruation, people with piles, or other causes of blood loss from the gut, such as hookworm infestation.
- Insufficient iron or certain vitamins (B12 and folic acid) in the diet: see *Nutrition*, section 1.1 for sources.
- Destruction of red cells or defective formation by the bone marrow and other blood-forming organs, caused by severe infections and drugs (such as sulphonamides, phenacetin and phenylbutazone).

What are the symptoms?

Paleness, excessive tiredness, fainting or giddiness and shortness of breath are all symptoms of anaemia. These may have other causes, however, including anxiety or depression as well as physical causes, so you should let the doctor diagnose and treat you. Heavy periods may be caused by anaemia, as well as causing anaemia.

How can it be prevented?

- A good balanced diet.
- Avoidance of unnecessary medication.
- Wear sandals or shoes to prevent being infected with hookworm which exist in wet muddy areas in warm climates.

How can it be treated?

See a doctor if you have these symptoms. By taking iron tablets you may be masking something that needs treatment. If you have very heavy periods you should take extra iron but see a doctor when you can.

Iron comes in many forms: in foods, such as green leafy vegetables; in iron syrups and tablets, sometimes mixed with vitamins. Vitamin C enhances its absorption from the stomach.

The suggested dosage for someone with heavy blood loss during periods is Ferrous sulphate 200mg, 1 tablet once, twice or up to 3 times daily or Ferrous gluconate and fumarate are good alternatives in the same dosage.

NOTES
- Iron in the above dosages will cause the stools to be black or dark coloured.
- It may also cause constipation in some; in others it may cause diarrhoea or nausea. If you experience these side effects then reduce the dose or stop taking the tablets and discuss the problem with a doctor.
- Overdosage with iron can cause deposits of iron to be laid down in the liver and other organs, causing damage, so beware of taking iron unless you know you need it.

ANGINA

What is it?
It is a tightness or pain felt across the chest, usually on the left, maybe up into the left side of the neck or into the left arm. It is brought on by exercise or by emotional stress, and relieved by rest. It may be associated with shortness of breath. Angina is very rare indeed in people below the age of 40.

What is the cause?
It may be due to 'furring up' of the blood-vessels supplying the heart, so that, when the heart is subjected to extra work, as in exercise, insufficient blood, and therefore oxygen, gets to the heart muscle (a bit like a 'stitch'). Angina could be the first warnings of a heart being 'overworked and underpaid', that is, not supplied with sufficient blood and oxygen!

What to do about it
You should see a doctor if you think you may have angina. Indigestion, anxiety, muscular strain and chest infections can cause similar pain, but you may need some investigation and treatment.

How can you prevent it developing?
Angina may be the result of a lifetime of eating the wrong foods, such as those high in cholesterol (see *Nutrition*, section 1.1) or of years of smoking. Changing your diet to a high-fibre, low-fat one by avoiding animal fats and reducing the amount of eggs and dairy produce you eat, eating fish one or more times a week and stopping smoking, will help to prevent any further development of some of the causes of angina, and may perhaps prevent later heart attacks.

ANXIETY AND TENSION

A feeling of tension is a normal, healthy response to danger or stress, and is part of the body's 'fight or flight' reaction. The danger or stress may be physical or emotional, and it is only when the anxiety persists with physical symptoms that it can become a problem or even a real illness.

The symptoms and the causes vary from person to person; the causes may be entirely understandable and natural, or may be so deep-seated and apparently unconnected to the present circumstances that it would take considerable skill by a doctor or counsellor to 'unearth' the cause.

Common physical symptoms of anxiety
- A more rapid heartbeat and respiratory rate than usual.
- A constant feeling of tension (see also *Pre-menstrual tension*, in section 5.3).
- Headaches and muscle tensions or aches.
- Sleep disturbances, such as early waking.
- Loss or increase of appetite.
- Recurrent indigestion.
- Increased sweating.
- Frequency of passing urine or loose frequent stools.

All these may have other causes too, but see further under *Stress*, section 1.3, for more details.

What to do
- If your circumstances make the causes obvious, try to understand and if possible deal with these.
- Find someone to talk things through with, or write to a trusted friend.
- Relaxation techniques, ensuring time off, learning occasionally to say 'no' may help.

See further under *Relaxation*, section 1.4.

If the symptoms or problems persist
See a doctor, who may examine you to ensure there are no physical causes for your symptoms. You may just need to talk and be reassured.

Sleeping tablets and tranquillizers
The doctor may offer these. Don't despise or fear them, but use them sensibly and in consultation with the doctor. A short course of sleeping tablets (perhaps every night for a week, or once or twice a week for longer) may just help you to cope with the day's demands and see things in proportion. Mild tranquillizers used during the day for a week or two may also help with the symptoms and break the pattern of your reactions. They can cause drowsiness, so avoid driving or

using machinery. **All sleeping tablets and tranquillizers are habit-forming and may be addictive if taken regularly**.

For advice about actual tranquillizers and sleeping tablets, see section 8.

NOTE
Tranquillizers should only be used under medical supervision for short-term problems on an occasional basis. They should not be used to deal with the normal stresses of life or to suppress or dull the grief which is a normal reaction to bereavement. This grief should be properly expressed if it is not to cause serious problems later.

APPENDICITIS

What is it?
An inflammation of the appendix, which is a small appendage on the intestines.

What are the symptoms?
- Severe abdominal pain starting around the upper or middle parts of the abdomen and moving to the lower right. The pain is usually continuous, and may be dull or sharp, and is worse when moving or coughing. There is tenderness on pressure over the right lower abdomen and it may be difficult to stand up straight.
- Loss of appetite, nausea and vomiting. The vomiting usually starts after the pain, and in small children may be more marked than the pain.
- Fever is usually present, though not high.
- Constipation for a day or two is common.

See also other causes of abdominal pain, but do not delay in seeking medical help if you suspect appendicitis.
NOTE
Abdominal pain with diarrhoea is not usually due to appendicitis.

What should you do?
- Take (or give) sips of water only.
- **Go to a doctor** or hospital as soon as possible if you think you or your child may have appendicitis: surgery may be necessary to remove the inflamed appendix.
- **Important**
  - do not take antibiotics
  - do not take laxatives
  - if symptoms are becoming worse quickly, do not delay, especially if you have any distance to go.

APPETITE

Loss of appetite

This occurs in a large number of conditions, and may be the first symptom of a developing infection, such as hepatitis. It may also be a sign of anxiety or depression, or of some chronic illness, especially if it is accompanied by loss of weight. If it persists you should see a doctor. It could be caused by something as simple as very warm, humid weather or a worm infestation.

Increased appetite

This could be just a sign of well-being or an increase in physical effort. However, some people eat more if they are anxious or depressed, just before periods, or when taking the contraceptive Pill. Occasionally an increased appetite with *loss* of weight can be a sign of an illness such as an over-active thyroid, or a tape-worm infection.

ARTHRITIS

What is it?

The word means inflammation of one or several joints. There are many causes for this condition, the most common being wear and tear over many years, the sort known as osteo-arthritis that older people often develop. Virus or bacterial infections, trauma such as a joint fracture, and general inflammatory conditions such as rheumatoid arthritis, are also causes.

Can it be prevented?

Since 'it' is not a single entity this is a difficult question to answer. In general terms the answer is probably not, but being more specific there are one or two situations where a little forethought may help in later years.

What you can do

● Install a head-rest on the driver and front passenger seats of your car which will protect your neck from a possible whiplash injury in case of accident. Whiplash injuries can cause problems with arthritis in the neck in later years.

● Learn to lift properly so that you do not constantly strain your back by lifting with it in the bent position. You should learn to lift from your hips and knees, keeping your back straight.

● If you develop severe pains and swelling **in several joints at once**, go to bed and rest, take 2 aspirin or paracetamol tablets every 4 hours and try to arrange to see a doctor within days or as soon as possible. This could be the beginning of one of the viral illnesses or one of the general inflammatory conditions, and your joints need to be protected by rest and the anti-inflammatory effect of the tablets. A bandage will help to support any severely painful joint.

- **If one joint swells**, becomes red and painful, rest it, take aspirin, 2 tablets 4-hourly, and arrange to see a doctor as soon as possible if it is not settling down within 24 hours. **If you have a temperature**, do not delay: you could have an infection inside the joint that requires immediate antibiotic treatment. A bandage will help to support the joint.

ASTHMA

What is it?
Difficulty in breathing, with a wheezing sound from the chest, caused by the small air tubes in the lungs going into spasm. The wheeze is often more noticeable when breathing out.

What causes it?
It is usually an allergic reaction, triggered by a variety of stresses:

- Specific allergens, such as pollens, fur, certain foods, some inhalants.
- Viral respiratory infections.
- In some people, exercise.
- In some people, emotional upsets.

Varieties
For some it starts in childhood with frequent episodes associated with colds and coughs; in some it is associated with exercise; and in some it comes on suddenly as an allergy.

What is the treatment?
Small children: see *Wheezing*, section 5.4. Exercise-induced in children and young adults: take the prescribed medication **regularly** unless the attacks are very rare.

The commonly-used medications are:

- **Ventolin** (salbutamol). As syrup, tablets or inhaler. Only useful to *dilate* the air tubes at the time of an attack, and should be used at the first sign of one. May also be used *just* before a period of exercise. It will only work if the Ventolin is carried on the breath *into* the lungs as you breathe in.
- **Intal** (sodium cromoglycate). Spinhaler or inhaler. Used **regularly** this will reduce or eliminate the number of attacks — it prevents the whole process starting. It will have *no* effect during an attack. Take 1 – 2 puffs 2 – 4 times a day, starting with 4 times and reducing to twice as the condition comes under control. Some Olympic runners use this.

● **Becotide** (Beclomethasone diproprionate). Inhaler, also for **regular** use. Contains a small dose of steroid which has a local effect, but not enough of a general effect to be serious when used as prescribed. This also should be taken in 1–2 puffs 2–4 times daily, starting with 4 and reducing as the condition comes under control.

All ages — due to specific allergies: avoid the cause if possible. Carry your Ventolin or other inhaler with you. If it is not possible to avoid the cause, **always** carry your Ventolin inhaler (or similar), and Piriton (or other antihistamine) tablets, and take a dose of each at the first sign of an attack or take regularly if so advised.

NOTE

Learn to use your inhaler correctly and do not exceed the recommended dose.

When to call a doctor or go to hospital

● When the measures previously mentioned are not helping.
● When the wheezing or tightness becomes more severe in spite of the usual treatment.
● When you begin to feel very tired or drowsy.
● If the wheezing is sudden, severe, and accompanied by swelling of the face, eyes or throat: **This needs immediate treatment by injection**. See *Allergy*.
● If the tightness in the chest is accompanied by a pain in the left chest, neck or arm.
● If you have a high temperature and are coughing up yellow or green phlegm.

What you can do

● Sit upright, leaning forward slightly with arms held over a chairback or 2 high pillows.
● Prop a child up with pillows.
● Steam inhalations sometimes help.
● Make sure you have used your inhaler correctly.

But do not delay in travelling to a hospital or calling a doctor if any of these symptoms develop. See further under *Asthma*, section 5.4.

ATHLETE'S FOOT

See *Skin problems*.

BACK-ACHE

Persistent, nagging low back-ache has a wide variety of causes, and the cause is not always obvious.

What are the commonest causes?

Tiredness, bad posture, being overweight, a soft bed, incorrect driving or working posture, high heels, constipation, lack of exercise, pre-menstrual or menstrual tension, period pain are all responsible for back-ache.

What you can do about it
● Correct these causes, where possible, by changing to lower heels, losing weight, doing back exercises or going swimming and so on.
● If the pain persists in spite of correction of any of the above possible causes, then you should be examined by a doctor. In women, for example, a new and persistent low back-ache might indicate some disease of the womb or Fallopian tubes (see also *Menstrual problems, Salpingitis*, section 5.3).

BACK PAIN
Severe, localized back pain also has a variety of causes.

What are the commonest causes?
Muscle strain, due to awkward twisting movements, or lifting a heavy object with a bent back, not only causes pain but can also cause a slipped disc.

What you can do about it
● If you have severe pain down a leg as well and the pain increases with coughing or sneezing, go to a doctor or hospital as soon as possible.

● If the pain is localized to one area only:
  − Lie flat on your back in bed (with a board under the mattress if the bed is soft, or with the mattress on the floor) with only 1 pillow under your head and a smaller pillow in the small of your back and under your knees. If your pain is not eased by this, lie in the most comfortable position.
  − Take aspirin, 2 tablets, or paracetamol, 2 tablets, every 4 hours.
  − Apply a hot-water bottle to the affected area, or a hot compress.
  − Gentle massage of the painful area might help too.
  − Gradually, over several days, increase the amount you do, and start gentle back-strengthening exercises. A muscle strain will take a week or two to clear up.
If the pain persists go to see a doctor.

NOTES
Influenza and any fever commonly causes back-ache and limb pains. Aspirin or paracetamol 4-hourly will help.
  Urinary tract infections can cause back-ache but are

usually accompanied by other symptoms.

BELL'S PALSY

What is it?
It is a sudden paralysis of one side of the face which is found usually upon waking. The face has a lopsided look, feels numb, and one eye will not close properly. Sometimes one side of the mouth droops or the face looks pulled over to one side. This is because the muscles on the paralysed side are weak or not working, so the stronger muscles pull the face over towards them. It is not the same thing as a stroke, and the person usually recovers completely.

What causes it?
It is probably caused by a virus infection, resulting in a swelling of the facial nerve where it passes through a bony canal. The compression due to the swelling causes the nerve to become paralysed.

What can be done about it?
It is important to ask a doctor to examine you to ensure there is no other cause for your paralysis. **The most important thing is to protect the eye**: if the eyelids will not close, the lining of the eye becomes dried out and damaged; this can lead to

infection and scarring which will interfere with vision. Protect the eye by:
● Artificial tear drops.
● Keeping a pad over it to keep it closed (or use Micropore tape).
A doctor should advise you if anything else needs to be done, and he should examine the eye regularly. He may prescribe:
● A course of steroid tablets to reduce the swelling and the severity of the paralysis. These are very powerful drugs and quite high doses are needed.
● Physiotherapy and gentle massage of the affected muscles.
Be patient: it usually takes 3–6 months to recover, but most people *do* recover. In the meantime, take great care of your eye.

BERIBERI

What is it?
It is an illness caused by a deficiency of thiamin (vitamin B1) in the diet. It tends to occur in people who have a very inadequate diet consisting mainly of, for example, polished rice (the vitamin B1 exists in the husks of rice). It also occurs in chronic alcoholics and in some severe illnesses, and occasionally in pregnancy if the diet is inadequate.

How can it be prevented?

- Ensure your diet includes wholegrain cereals, peas, beans and nuts; also milk, liver or kidneys if you are not a vegetarian.
- If possible, eat brown rice (that is, with the husks) rather than polished rice. This provides you with fibre as well as vitamin B1 and other nutrients.
- Avoid becoming an alcoholic.

See further under *Nutrition*, section 1.1 for more details.

What are the symptoms?

Early symptoms include:

- Excessive tiredness, and irritability.
- Memory loss.
- Lack of appetite.
- Constipation (though this may be more to do with the lack of fibre in your diet).
- Tingling in the toes with burning of the soles of the feet (probably at night).
- Calf muscle cramps and leg pains.

Later symptoms include neurological and heart problems and need to be diagnosed and treated by a doctor.

What is the treatment?

- Improving the diet.
- Vitamin B1 in doses estimated according to the severity of the illness.

'BLACK EYE'
See *Eye problems*.

BLOOD POISONING

What is it?

It is a bacterial infection spreading through the bloodstream from a focus of infection such as an infected cut or a tooth abscess. Sometimes it is caused by a toxin produced by the bacteria that is being carried around in the circulation.

What are the symptoms?

- Chills with shivering and feeling cold however many blankets you cover yourself with.
- Usually high 'spiking' temperatures which go up quickly and often drop again quickly with a lot of sweating.

NOTE

There may be other symptoms, too, related to the severity and source of the infection. The shivering and fever may be very like a malaria infection, and if you live in a malarious area this would be the first thing that would have to be excluded by blood tests. See further under *Malaria*, section 6.

What is the treatment?

This depends on the cause, so

a diagnosis should first be made. You should see a doctor as soon as possible. This type of fever is *not* something you should treat yourself unless you are sure it is caused by malaria. If you treat the symptoms as if they are caused by malaria but they do not clear within 24–36 hours on the anti-malaria treatment, you *must* travel to see a doctor. See *What to do on a journey to hospital*, section 3.2.

BLOOD PRESSURE

What is it?
It is a combination of the force with which the heart pumps the blood around the circulation (systolic pressure) and the resistance or elasticity in the smaller blood-vessels of the system (diastolic). The normal ranges are 100–140mm of mercury for systolic and 60–80mm for diastolic. The blood pressure *rises* when the small vessels lose their elasticity (as in atherosclerosis) and the heart has to work harder to pump the blood around the circulatory system. Blood pressure usually goes up to some extent with age. When it is persistently found to be above the normal range for your age it is called *hypertension*.

What causes it to rise?
A combination of several factors are usually involved.
Temporarily:
● Exercise, emotional stress and fear — this is a normal response with only a small rise, and usually causes no problem.
● Some people have a 'labile hypertension', which means the blood pressure goes up and down very easily in response to some temporary stress.
● Pregnancy, sometimes; the contraceptive Pill, sometimes.
Permanently:
● Being overweight, smoking.
● High salt intake may contribute.
● 'Furring up' of the arteries as in atherosclerosis (possibly associated with high cholesterol intake).
● Some kidney diseases.
● In most cases no cause can be found, although there may be an inherited tendency to high blood pressure.

Can one avoid developing hypertension?
Not always, but it is wise to avoid the factors which are known to be associated with it. So, for example:
● Don't smoke.
● Avoid becoming or remaining overweight.
● Avoid an excessive salt intake.
● Avoid an excessive cholesterol intake (foods

containing animal fats, butter, cheese and egg yolk), and increase your fibre intake (foods such as beans, cereals, and vegetables) which reduces the absorption of cholesterol from the gut, and also the absorption of carbohydrate. Eat fish once or more per week. The fat that fish contains is of the poly-unsaturated variety, and seems to have a protective effect, helping to prevent the development of blood pressure and heart problems. See further under *Nutrition*, section 1.1.

What are the symptoms?

Usually there are none, but some people experience severe, continuing headaches, and older people may experience nosebleeds. Tiredness, breathlessness and visual disturbance may also be associated with a rise in blood pressure.

What is the treatment?

This is usually preceded by some investigations to establish, if possible, the cause. The treatment is usually with tablets (which may have to be continued for life), with regular blood pressure checks, and advice about diet and smoking.

BOILS AND ABSCESSES

See also *Acne*, *Dental problems*, *Skin problems*.

What is a boil?

A boil is caused by an infection in the root (or follicle) of a hair. Several may develop at once, and they are most likely to occur in areas which are usually moist or where the skin is particularly greasy. When a lot of grease (or sebum, which is produced by a gland in the root of the hair) builds up, the follicle may become blocked; bacteria then cause an infection and pus develops inside the follicle which swells and becomes painful. It may eventually burst but is best left alone.

What can you do to prevent boils developing?

● Keep the skin as clean as possible with daily or more frequent washing with soap and water; ensure the soap has been properly rinsed off.

A good moisturizer will help to stop the skin of your face becoming too dry, but avoid very greasy ones.

● If you think a boil is beginning to develop, *do not squeeze it*! This only makes matters worse. Dab it with eau-de-Cologne or TCP or similar antiseptic using sterile or clean cotton wool.

How to treat boils

- Apply TCP or similar antiseptic.
- Do not squeeze!
- Bathe with hot water, which sometimes 'brings them out' or helps them heal.
- Occasionally, if boils are constantly recurring or large and painful, a course of Oxytetracycline 250mg 4 times daily for 5 days may help.

If you have access to a doctor, and the boils keep recurring in spite of the above treatment, ask for an examination of your urine for sugar, and if possible, a nose swab to be cultured, as the bacteria causing the boils may be harboured in the nose.

What is an abscess?

This is a much larger collection of pus than a boil; it is usually much more painful and often accompanied by recurrent high rises in temperature. An abscess can occur anywhere in the body: such as the root of a tooth, in the tissue under the skin, in a muscle, in the abdominal cavity.

What is the treatment?

The collection of pus has to be let out, and this usually involves some surgery, so you must arrange to see a doctor as soon as possible (or a dentist if it is a tooth abscess: he may have to remove the tooth). Antibiotics are also sometimes prescribed:

seek medical advice.

BRONCHITIS

What is it?

This is an inflammation of the air tubes in the lungs, often caused by a bacterial infection following on from a common cold or influenza.

What are the symptoms?

A cough with the production of yellow or green, nasty-tasting phlegm (sputum), fever and tiredness or weakness.

What is the treatment?

- Rest.
- If you can do so, see a doctor, who will probably prescribe antibiotics. If a doctor is not available, see section 8 for advice about antibiotics and cough mixtures.
- Cough mixtures suppress the cough and should only be taken at night so that you (and others) can sleep. The cough helps to get rid of the infected phlegm, so is useful unless it is tiring you out too much.
- Steam inhalations twice a day (on their own or with Vick, Friar's Balsam, Karvol, or similar) help to loosen the phlegm and clear the chest.

It usually takes a week or so to clear and may leave you feeling tired for another couple of weeks.

NOTE
If you have any pain in the lower chest or in the back on coughing or breathing deeply then you should arrange to see a doctor as soon as possible. You can start treatment with steam inhalations.

BRUCELLOSIS

This is also known as undulant fever because it has a typically recurring pattern of fever, 'undulating' up and down.

How is it caught?

It is caught through drinking milk of cattle or goats infected with the organism, or from direct contact with the blood or excreta of infected animals, or from inhaling infected dust. Cattle, goats, sheep and pigs are the animals most commonly infected.

How can it be prevented?

- Milk should be boiled or pasteurized, and meat cooked to 'well done'.
- Protective clothing and spectacles should be used by those working with infected herds.
- It is possible to immunize animals against brucellosis, but not, so far, people.

What are the symptoms?

High, swinging fever with chills and sweating, often very similar to malaria, but lasting much longer.

What is the treatment?

Any fever which lasts for longer than 3 or 4 days, or which recurs, should be investigated and treated by a doctor: this is not something for self-medication. (See section 3.2 for advice about what to do if you have to travel to a hospital or a doctor.)

NOTE
If you live in a malarious area, see section 6 for treatment of malaria. However, if the fever does not clear within 24 – 36 hours of starting the treatment against malaria, you must make the effort to be seen by a doctor.

BUGS AND SMALL BEASTIES

This includes bed-bugs, fleas, ticks, chiggers, scabies, head and body lice.

BED-BUGS

These creatures live in cracks in walls, floors, and in furniture, blankets and mattresses. They respond to human warmth and seek out the source in search of a blood meal. They bite and have an objectionable smell, but are not necessarily disease carriers.

How to get rid of them

- Put bedclothes, mattresses and furniture out in the sun for several hours each day.

• Spray walls, floors and furniture with DDT, HCH (Gammexane) or organophosphorous insecticides such as malathion or diazinon. Unfortunately bed-bugs often develop resistance to DDT and HCH. Remember that the insecticides may also be dangerous to people, especially the organophosphorous ones, and DDT is dangerous to animals.

How to treat the bites

They are itchy, but try to scratch as little as possible to avoid them becoming infected. Anthisan Cream may soothe (but do not use too often or too regularly as you may develop a sensitivity reaction to it). Savlon, TCP or a similar antiseptic will also soothe and help to prevent infection, as will eau-de-Cologne. The itchiness will usually settle in 2–3 days.

CHIGGERS (or Jiggers)

These are ticks, mites or other insects which have burrowed into the skin (often the feet) and caused a local swelling and infection. Sometimes an egg is laid in the burrow and a small larva develops in there.

How to treat an infected chigger

• A strong alcohol such as surgical spirit or antiseptic solution may help to kill off the 'chigger'. Sometimes it is then possible to 'dig it out' with a needle sterilized by holding the point in a flame for a minute.

• Soak the foot in antiseptic or salt solution for 10 minutes morning and evening, dry it and apply antiseptic cream or powder to the sore. Do this daily until it heals.

• If the area around the 'chigger' is red and swollen, and there are red lines going from it up the leg, you may need a course of antibiotics. If a doctor is available ask his advice.

• If you do not have access to a doctor, take a course of Penicillin tablets (250mg every 6 hours for 7 days). See section 8 for further advice about antibiotics and alternatives if you cannot take Penicillin.

NOTE

If the inflamed red lines do not start to disappear within 2–3 days of starting the antibiotic, or if you start to run a fever, or if the glands in your groin or armpit on the affected side become swollen and painful, you *must* seek out a doctor or travel to a hospital. Continue to take the antibiotics and apply the antiseptic to the sore while you wait for further treatment. See section 3.2 for advice about what to do on the journey.

FLEAS

Fleas jump from person to person, or from animals such as cats and dogs. They bite and suck blood, leaving irritating red marks, often in several clusters or in a line up a leg or an arm. Some fleas are disease carriers.

How to avoid them or get rid of them

- Ensure your cats, dogs, or other furry pets, are free of fleas by using flea-collars, or flea powders to kill them off. (Beware of DDT which may be dangerous — especially to cats.)
- Fleas may hide in furniture or clothes, so put furniture and bedclothes out in the sun for several hours, and wash clothes and hang these out in the sun. If ironing, make a point of ironing the seams thoroughly as fleas hide from the sun in such places.
- Insecticides sprayed in the house (as for bed-bugs) may help.

How to treat the bites

See *Bed-bugs*.

TICKS AND MITES

These bury their biting parts in the skin while sucking blood. When they have taken their fill they will remove these and depart, leaving a similar itchy red mark or swelling to that caused by a bed-bug or a flea. There are several varieties: a hard-backed tick lives in long grass and may carry tick typhus; a soft-backed variety inhabits human dwellings and may carry relapsing fever.

How to avoid and get rid of them

- Use residual insecticides such as HCH (Gammexane) in the house from time to time.
- Dust your feet and ankles with sulphur or DDT powder (if your skin is not sensitive to it) before going out into forest or grass lands where you know ticks exist.
- If you find one on you do *not* try to remove it forcibly. It will only leave its biting part behind in your skin, causing irritation and probably infection. It has to be induced to let go of its bite by putting a drop of alcohol, oil or paraffin on it.

How to treat the bites

- A piece of ice held against the bite will reduce the irritation.
- Treat the bite as for flea or bed-bug bites, and see also Infected bites or Chiggers.

SCABIES

This is caused by tiny mites which burrow under the skin, causing an itchy rash which is commonly seen between the fingers, on the inside of the wrists and up the arms, and also on other parts of the body. The mites are passed on by close personal contact with someone who is infected. The itchiness is particularly intense when you are warm.

How to avoid scabies

- Avoid close personal skin-to-skin contact with anyone you do not know very well, and especially if the person has an itchy rash anywhere. Bedclothes may also harbour the mites, so sleeping in someone else's dirty bedclothes may also infect you.
- Maintain good personal hygiene by bathing regularly, wearing clean clothes and hanging the bedclothes out in the sun in warm climates.

How to treat scabies

- Although this is itchy, scratching should be avoided as this may break the skin surface so that the tunnels or burrows in the skin become infected with bacteria. The mites themselves also carry infection into the skin.
- Bath in clean warm water with soap, scrubbing your skin well with a soft brush or a flannel (which will need boiling afterwards to get rid

of the mites that have come away with the surface skin cells).
- An infusion of Neem leaves (or similar leaves with antiseptic properties) may be used to wash yourself with. The Neem leaves themselves can be used to scrub the skin.
- Dry yourself on a towel kept just for you. Wash the towel and hang out in the sun.
- Sulphur ointment may then be applied to all the areas that have any spots or rash. This should be done daily until the rash is gone.

OR

- Make up a mixture of 15 parts Vaseline and 1 part Lindane (gamma benzene hexachloride) and apply this to all the affected parts once a week until the infection has cleared. Bath daily, even after applying the Lindane/Vaseline mixture.

OR

- Apply a lotion of Benzyl benzoate to the whole body (except face and neck) after bathing as above. This should be done 3 times at 12 hourly intervals if the infection is severe; if mild, once may be enough.

HEAD AND BODY LICE
(or crab lice)
The human louse is a small creature which lays many eggs (nits) at a time on the

hair or on clothing fibres. The adult may bite and cause severe itching which in turn gives rise to skin infections from the scratching which results. Lice may carry several diseases, including typhus and poliomyelitis if their bites have drawn blood from their victims. They are extremely common, especially among school children who pass them on to each other as they play together. 'Crab lice' live in pubic hair and are passed on by close physical contact.

How to avoid them

Avoid close mixing with those who are infected. This is clearly difficult for children and may not be possible.

How to get rid of head lice

Do *not* cut off your hair: it is quite unnecessary and can cause a great deal of embarrassment and difficulty. There are several different treatments: avoid getting any of them into the eyes:

EITHER

● Soak the hair in hot vinegar and water for half an hour to kill the nits, then comb through thoroughly with a fine-toothed comb.

OR

● Shampoo with Prioderm (malathion) or Carylderm (carbaryl) or Lorexane (gamma benzene hexachloride) — leave to dry for 12 hours, then shampoo and comb through thoroughly with a fine-toothed comb to remove the remaining nits. Repeat as necessary 1 week later.

OR

● Use a mixture of Lindane 1 part to 10 parts of water, mixed with an ordinary shampoo to make a lather. Comb hair thoroughly with a fine-toothed comb to remove the nits. Repeat after 1 week.

For crab lice use either of the last 2 treatments, avoiding the more sensitive areas. Take a bath after applying the treatment.

'BURSITIS'

See *Joint pains*.

CHEST PAIN

Pain in the chest has a variety of causes, the commonest ones being:

Indigestion

A burning discomfort or pain up the central part of the chest and upper abdomen is known as indigestion or heartburn. It usually occurs within an hour of eating or because the stomach is empty. See a doctor if it comes on suddenly and severely. See *Indigestion*. A sharp, sudden pain lasting for a second is often due to wind.

Colds and Chest Infections

A dry cough is often accompanied by pain in the upper, middle part of the chest which is caused by inflammation of the large air tube, the trachea. There is often a sore throat or a hoarse voice. Aspirin or paracetamol, cough mixture and hot drinks may help. See *Colds and coughs*.

Muscle Pains

These are caused by coughing, or straining when lifting a heavy object, or an awkward movement. They are usually made worse by movement. Rest, aspirin or paracetamol and patience are the only treatment, but a hot water bottle and some massage may help to ease the pain.

Angina

See a doctor if you think you have angina. See *Angina*.

Heart Attacks

These are experienced as a very severe gripping pain across the chest from the left, accompanied by breathlessness, a change in colour, often a great sense of fear, and perhaps loss of consciousness. A doctor or hospital is needed very urgently. See *Heart Attacks*.

Pneumonia and Pleurisy

There is a severe pain in the lower part of the chest usually towards the sides and back. It is accompanied by fever and the person will appear quite ill. Deep breathing and coughing makes the pain worse. Anyone with this complaint should be seen and examined by a doctor as soon as possible: it should not be treated without expert help. Don't delay in the hope that it will 'go away'. See *Pneumonia*, *Pleurisy*.

For women taking the contraceptive Pill

Sudden pain in the chest, usually accompanied by a dry cough 'out of the blue', *must* always be investigated by a doctor. Stop taking the Pill and see a doctor at once. It could be caused by a blood clot that has 'lodged' in the lungs.
NOTE
Any unexplained pain in the chest, especially if it affects your breathing, must be checked by a doctor as soon as possible.

'CHINESE RESTAURANT SYNDROME'

What is it?

Monosodium glutamate, often used in Chinese cooking and in many pre-packaged convenience foods to give a meaty flavour, causes burning sensations in the body if taken in sufficient quantities, and a feeling of pressure in the face and chest pain. The 'dose' required to produce these side-effects differs widely in individuals.

What is the treatment?
Stop eating foods containing monosodium glutamate! The symptoms clear up as the body gets rid of it.

CIRRHOSIS

What is it?
It is a condition of the liver in which irregular patches of fibrosis or 'scarring' of the liver tissue takes place as a result of 'injury' or damage to the liver. The severity of the cirrhosis depends on the severity of the damage, and there is no treatment to cure it.

What causes it?
It has a number of causes, although it is also possible to be born with it (congenital cirrhosis). The causes include, among other things, long-term regular intake of too much alcohol, some viral illnesses, and poisoning with some toxic substances.

How can it be prevented?
● Avoid over-indulgence in alcohol.
● If you travel in countries where hepatitis (especially the hepatitis B variety) is common, ensure personal and food hygiene, clean water supply, avoid having injections by anyone you do not trust to use sterile needles, and have the gamma-globulin injections (protection against hepatitis A), and hepatitis B vaccine if advised to do so.

'COLD SORES'

What are 'cold sores'?
They are small patches on or near the lips or nose which start off feeling itchy or sore, then develop tiny blisters. These may 'weep' clear fluid and eventually crust over. The process usually takes about 10 days, but may be longer or shorter.

What causes them?
They are caused by a virus (Herpes simplex) which, once it has entered the cells of the skin, may remain dormant, and from time to time when you are under stress or have some other illness, causes the typical 'cold sore'. These are likely to recur over many years.

How can they be avoided?
● By avoiding close physical contact with someone who has a cold sore: don't kiss!
● Eat a good diet full of

vitamin C and keep as fit as possible.

How can they be treated?

- Dab the irritated patch of skin with TCP, eau-de-Cologne or other antiseptic, 2 or 3 times a day. Use Vaseline to soften, and cover.
- Avoid touching or rubbing as this will spread the infection and maybe cause bacteria to also infect the area.
- There are now anti-viral creams and lotions which may reduce the severity of the attack if applied at the first signs of a cold sore developing. These anti-viral agents are often only available on a doctor's prescription, and are very expensive.

The two commonly used agents are:

Idoxyuridine (Herpid)

Acyclovir (Zovirax)

COLDS AND COUGHS

All of us experience these from time to time. They are usually caused by viruses, and you will probably take a week to recover if it is not treated with anything and 7 days if it is!

An uncomplicated cold is one where you have a runny or very 'stuffed up' nose, probably a sore throat, a heavy head and perhaps a dry, irritating cough. There is no temperature rise usually, or only a slight one.

What you can do

- Take 1 or 2 tablets of aspirin or paracetamol to ease headaches and sore throats.
- Drink plenty of hot soothing drinks, such as lemon and honey with hot water.
- Take a cough mixture if the cough is very bothersome.
- Take a decongestant or do inhalations (see *Common drugs*, section 8).

Complications

Colds may lead on to secondary bacterial infections, such as sinusitis or bronchitis which may need antibiotics. See further under *Sinusitis* and *Bronchitis*.

COLIC

This is a wave or spasm of abdominal pain which lasts a minute or so, then goes off, leaving you feeling faint and a bit sick. It often precedes diarrhoea. If you do not have diarrhoea, and the pain continues to recur, especially if it is accompanied by a rise in temperature or vomiting, see a doctor as soon as possible. Some small babies appear to get 'colic' in the first 2 – 3 months: see *Colic*, section 5.4.

COLITIS, ULCERATIVE

What is it?
It is a condition of the large intestine (the colon) in which the lining becomes inflamed causing severe diarrhoea with blood and mucus. It can be very similar to amoebic dysentery, but is not caused by an infection. It may run in the family, and may start at any age.

How is it treated?
This needs diagnosis and long-term treatment and follow-up by a specialist in intestinal problems. The treatment involves medication and diet.

CONJUNCTIVITIS
See *Eye problems*.

CONSTIPATION
It used to be said that it was quite normal and healthy to open your bowels only 2 or 3 times a week. However, we now realize that many illnesses are caused by or related to constipation. Some of these include piles (haemorrhoids), varicose veins, diverticulitis and maybe other more serious problems.

Establishing good habits
It is a good idea to establish a pattern of good daily bowel movements from an early age. This is *not* best done, however, by an obsessional 'checking' or an absolutely clock-work system: it is best done by ensuring an adequate intake of fibre or roughage in our diets from early days.

Fibre is the unrefined, normally undigested, parts of cereals, such as wheat or maize, beans, fruit and vegetables. Fruit and vegetables alone do not provide the full amount required. It is a good idea only to eat wholemeal bread, for example, and to encourage your child to eat muesli and other 'whole' cereals, or bran-cereals, as well as daily portions of fresh fruit and vegetables. As soon as children develop teeth, they can be given pieces of apple or carrots or crispbread to chew on, rather than biscuits and sweetened foods: this will help prevent them developing a 'sweet tooth' and eating only refined foods which are bad for the teeth as well as the bowels.

If you have had problems with constipation for years and been used to taking laxatives such as Senokot, your gut needs to go through a process of 're-education'. This may take several weeks. Try to eat *at least* 2–3 tablespoons of bran (the dry, flaky kind) every day mixed with milk and another cereal; or mix it with soup, gravy, stews or with yoghurt.

Bran takes on the taste of whatever you mix it with. Eat only wholemeal bread; increase your intake of fresh fruit, vegetables and beans, and eat prunes or other dried fruits if available.

It will take a week or two of persevering with this before you notice much difference, though you may find you feel a bit 'bloated' and 'windy' during the initial weeks. Once you have achieved a change (for the better, hopefully) you will need to adjust your fibre intake to what is needed to give you 1 or 2 daily soft, large stools without any need to strain.

If your constipation persists in spite of the above, see a doctor for further advice.

NOTE
Increasing your fibre intake will also help you lose weight as it tends to 'fill you up' more, reduces cholesterol and carbohydrate absorption from your gut, and stops you feeling hungry as quickly as you tend to after a meal high in refined carbohydrates such as white flour, polished rice and sugar.

CONTRACEPTION

This means the prevention of pregnancy. There are basically 4 methods: natural, barrier, the coil or intra-uterine device (IUCD) and the Pill. Newer methods, such as hormone implants, are being developed.

Natural

● The withdrawal method is the withdrawal of the penis from the vagina just before ejaculation. It requires split-second timing and a lot of self-control. It is unreliable and can cause a lot of emotional strain.

● The calendar method involves calculating the time of ovulation each month and avoiding intercourse around this time. Again, this is not very reliable unless you have absolutely regular periods and are able to abstain from sexual intercourse for anything up to 14 days in any one month. The 'safe period' can be complicated to calculate, but if you are well motivated it can be successful, especially if combined with the temperature method.

● The temperature method also involves avoiding intercourse around the time of ovulation. The normal body temperature rises by about 0.3°C (0.6°F) at the time of ovulation, and remains at the higher level until the onset of the period. The early morning temperature has to be taken regularly before getting up or drinking anything. Intercourse should be avoided from 2 days before ovulation to 3 days after. This method is successful for some, but the temperature rise can be very difficult to assess and even experts make mistakes! It is more accurate if used together with the calendar method.

- The cervical mucus method also avoids intercourse around the time of ovulation. The mucus normally secreted by the cervix (the neck of the womb) becomes clear and jelly-like, rather like egg-white, at the time of ovulation and remains so for a couple of days. It is quite different from the discharge resulting from infection, or the normal mucus secretion at other times. It is more like the discharge produced by sexual stimulation. Women can become very expert at recognizing the change. Some women also get a pain in their right or left side for 24 hours or so at the actual time of ovulation, and this can be a further guide to the best time to avoid sexual intercourse to prevent pregnancy.

All these methods take a high degree of motivation and self-awareness.

NOTE

After intercourse, the sperm can survive for up to 72 hours in the womb. It is therefore important not only to avoid sexual intercourse for 72 hours after ovulation, but also 72 hours before, if fertilization is not to take place.

Barrier methods

These include the condom, sponges, diaphragms and caps. The condom or 'sheath', is the most popular, and provides 97–98% protection alone, or used together with spermicidal cream or jelly, provides 99% protection. (See glossary for use.)

These methods will also give a certain amount of protection against sexually-transmitted infections, and use of the sheath may protect against cancer of the neck of the womb (cervical cancer).

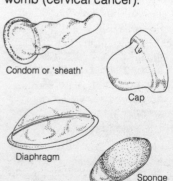

Condom or 'sheath'

Cap

Diaphragm

Sponge

The intra-uterine contraceptive device

The IUCD or coil has been widely used and is very acceptable for many women.

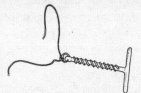

The coil has to be inserted by a doctor: some can then remain in place for years; others (of the copper variety) need changing every 2 to 3 years. However, there are some disadvantages:

- Some women develop heavy periods and cramping pains.
- Some women develop infections such as salpingitis, which can block the Fallopian tubes permanently, causing infertility.
- It is only about 97% effective.
- It probably works by preventing implantation of the fertilized ovum, and some people feel this is similar to an abortion.

'The Pill'

There are two varieties of oral contraceptive: the combined Pill, containing oestrogen and progestagen, and the progestagen only Pill. The first gives almost 100% protection if taken regularly, as it works by preventing ovulation. The second works by changing the cervical mucus so that it becomes hostile to the sperm, and is not quite so effective.

Most women have no problems on the Pill, but there are a small number who do. The main problems on the combined contraceptive Pill are as follows.

Not serious, but fairly common:

- An increased tendency to thrush or other vaginal or urinary infections.
- Weight gain due to an increased appetite.
- Depression or irritability, breast tenderness, and nausea, especially in the first month or so of taking it.

More serious, but very rare:

- A rise in blood pressure — which should be checked every 3–6 months while you are taking the contraceptive Pill.
- Deep vein thrombosis and embolism: see under *Phlebitis* and *Thrombophlebitis* for details of symptoms and treatment.
- A few women have problems conceiving for some months or longer when they stop taking the Pill.
- It is best to avoid conceiving until 3 months have elapsed after 'coming off' the Pill, as it is possible for it to affect the foetus.
- There is some evidence that cervical and breast cancer

may be associated with taking the Pill.

The Progesterone-only Pill has fewer side-effects, but may cause irregular bleeding; you should have the same check-ups as for the combined Pill.

Check-ups needed when taking the Pill

● Weight and blood pressure every 3–6 months.
● Breasts every 12 months.
● Cervical smear (PAP test) every 3 years, or more often if you have any problems with bleeding or have a history of genital Herpes infection.

You should not take the Pill if:

● You have a history of high blood pressure.
● You have a history of thrombophlebitis, or severe varicose veins or blood-clotting problems.
● You have a history of hepatitis or liver problems.
● There is a history of diabetes in the family.
● You are very overweight.
● You smoke and are over 35–40 years of age.

You should take it only after you have been examined by a doctor and your family and personal medical history has been checked. Do check that your Pill does not have a higher dose of oestrogen than 50 micrograms. Make sure you have a cervical, or PAP, smear

done at least every 3 years. This will detect cervical cancer in the early stages.

NOTE

If you develop diarrhoea and/or vomiting, the Pill may not be absorbed and you will not be protected that month. Beware also of some antibiotics and other medications which may interfere with the Pill. Check with the doctor.

New developments in contraception

A great deal of research is going on in this field, and many interesting possibilities are being tried out. Among these possibilities are the following:

● Improved spermicides which are longer acting.
● Improved IUCDs which release minute amounts of hormone and may last for up to 10 years.
● After-sex pills with high doses of hormones which have to be started within 72 hours of intercourse: used at present only in emergencies, as after rape.
● Once-a-month pills.
● Hormone nasal sprays.
● Silicone 'plugs' for the Fallopian tubes in women, and sperm tubes in men.
● Vaccines: probably still a long way to go as there are many technical difficulties.
● A Pill for men, or hormone creams, implants, and injections.

CONVULSIONS

See also *Febrile Convulsions in Childhood*, section 5.4 and *Epilepsy*, later in this section.

What is a convulsion?

A convulsion, or fit, is a sudden, uncontrollable, rhythmical jerking, usually of the whole body, but sometimes of only a limb. It is accompanied by a temporary loss of consciousness and followed by a period of drowsiness. There may be difficulty with breathing (this returns to normal once the convulsion stops), groaning sounds, grinding of teeth and incontinence of urine.

What to do if someone has a convulsion

1 Ease breathing by turning patient on one side or on front with face to one side and by loosening neck-tie or collar.
2 Control, but do not restrain forcibly. Ensure patient is on the floor or on a sofa or bed, with no hard or sharp edges nearby.
3 If you have a wooden spoon handy and the teeth become unclenched long enough, put this between the teeth to prevent the tongue being bitten — but watch your own fingers! Don't waste time on this unless immediately to hand.

4 In a child, the cause may be a high temperature: **get the temperature down by tepid sponging**. Strip patient and wet all over with water, and allow to dry off in the air.
5 Send someone to call a doctor if this is the first time the person has had a fit, or take to a hospital once the fit is over. If you do not know the person's past history, an examination should be carried out as soon as possible.
6 Meanwhile, stay with the person until the convulsion stops, ensuring that there is no obvious obstruction to breathing. Make a note of how long the convulsion lasts.
7 Once the convulsion has stopped make patient comfortable on one side or half-front ('recovery position') and allow sleep and gradual recovery. The person may be dazed for a while afterwards.

CYSTITIS

What is cystitis?

This is a bacterial infection of the urine, affecting the bladder. If the infection also involves the tubes to the kidneys, or the kidneys themselves, such words as pyelitis or pyelonephritis may be used: collectively any of these infections are known as urinary tract infections or UTIs.

What are the symptoms?
Cystitis involves:
- Passing small quantities of urine very frequently.
- Burning or stinging when passing urine.
- Sometimes the urine may have an unusual smell, or become cloudy or pink (this last is if there is any bleeding).
- Sometimes, lower abdominal discomfort, and general malaise.

Other symptoms, which develop if the infection is spreading to, or starting in the kidneys, include:
- Pain and tenderness in the waist area, towards the back or in the sides.
- Fever, sometimes with shivering attacks and vomiting.

What is the treatment?
- Drink about double your normal quantities to 'wash out the system' and 'dilute' the concentration of the bacteria.
- Mix 1–2 teaspoons of bicarbonate of soda in a glass of water and drink this 2 or 3 times daily, which may help by altering the acidity of the urine and making the bugs feel less welcome!
- If the symptoms are not clearing up within 24 hours or you are developing a temperature or pain in your back, you should, if possible, see a doctor, as a urine test would be a good idea before starting treatment. If not possible, take a *full* course of *Septrin, 2 tablets twice a day, for 10 days, or *Amoxil (or Ampicillin) 500mg, 8-hourly for 10 days. Don't stop after 3–4 days because you are feeling better: complete the course, as recurrences occur much more frequently if you do not, and the bacteria are likely to develop resistance.

NOTE
Septrin=Co trimoxazole
            +Trimethoprim
            +Sulphamethoxazoe
Amoxil=Amoxycillin (Ampicillin is similar)
Both these are expensive, and some people are allergic to them. Other alternatives are:
Nitrofurantoin 100mg
1 tablet×4, 6-hourly
Nalidixic acid 500mg
2 tablets×4, 6-hourly
Keflex=Cephalexin 500mg×3, 8-hourly
All should be taken for 10 days.

DEAFNESS
See *Hearing problems*

DENTAL HEALTH

Many dental problems can be prevented by adequate cleaning of teeth and a healthy diet.

What is meant by 'adequate cleaning'?

Ideally, teeth should be cleaned within 10 minutes of every meal, as the action of bacteria from the food debris takes place very rapidly. The bacteria excrete an acid which eats into the tooth substance. If cleaning after each meal is not possible, the teeth should at least be cleaned after breakfast and after the last thing you eat or drink at night.

How do I know if I'm cleaning my teeth properly?

Brush each tooth individually for about 10 seconds, remembering to clean all sides. Avoid side-to-side brushing, as this can cause areas of sensitive 'erosion'. A tooth-brush with a small head (a child's toothbrush, or one especially designed for this purpose) will make it easier for you to reach the last molars. Look in the mirror to check that you have done a thorough job. Once in 24 hours, finish by running Dental Floss between each tooth, and massaging the gums with dental sticks. It is removing the 'plaque' that is important. If it is too impractical to clean your teeth after each meal, finish the meal with some fibrous food, such as an apple or carrot, or an unsweetened drink. If you are in a remote area where toothpaste is hard to obtain, or if you are without toothbrush or paste for some reason, ash or salt make a good substitute, and can be applied with the end of a stick frayed by chewing it!

What about diet?

Have a well-balanced diet (see section 1.1), avoiding too many sweets, biscuits, cakes, buns, fizzy drinks and other carbohydrates, especially when you can't clean your teeth afterwards. Try to avoid encouraging a 'sweet tooth' in a child, for instance, by giving unsweetened drinks right from the start. Give your children washed fruit or raw vegetables to eat instead of sweets. Keep a 'sweet box', if necessary, which they can have once a day, at a set time, and clean their teeth immediately afterwards.

Fluoride tablets and other similar measures, such as topical applications of fluoride, fluoride mouthwashes, or fissure sealing, are only effective when used in conjunction with good diet and tooth-cleaning. An excess of fluoride can cause a brownish discolouration of the enamel of the teeth so ensure you are not taking tablets if fluoride is added to the water you drink.

Sometimes a child's new teeth appear crooked and feel painful: very often this will improve as he grows, particularly in the lower jaw. If you are doubtful, the teeth should be checked in case orthodontic treatment is necessary. The erupting new teeth can cause pressure and soreness, and a dose of aspirin or paracetamol may be necessary. Wisdom teeth can cause pain, even if they are erupting normally. Frequent hot salt-water mouthwashes, with aspirin for the pain, will ease discomfort until you can report it to your dentist. This usually occurs in the 20 to 30 age group.

Sensitive teeth

'Sensodyne' and 'Emoform' toothpastes contain an ingredient which coats the teeth, thus protecting the sensitive areas. However, once started, these toothpastes should be used exclusively: their effectiveness is lost if another brand of toothpaste is used, as it will remove the protective coating.

TOOTHACHE

What are the causes?

Pain in or around a tooth is usually caused by a hole, an abscess or gum disease.

A hole

This is caused by the action of bacteria in the plaque that forms on teeth. Their action 'burns' a hole in the enamel, then the bacteria enter the deeper layers of enamel causing them to become rotten or carious. When the hole reaches the pulp or nerve part in the centre, the nerve becomes inflamed and soon starts to ache or hurt. The tooth becomes sensitive to hot and cold foods or drink, or to acid or sweet things.

An abscess

When the nerve or pulp becomes infected it may die causing an abscess. This is a collection of pus and dead material. The pain then becomes more continuous, severe and throbbing, and it hurts to bite on the tooth. As the abscess grows, the gum around it, and later the face, may swell.

Gum disease

This is also known as pyorrhoea. It is caused by infection and inflammation with swelling and soreness of the gums. Pockets form between the gum and the teeth. Debris collecting here becomes infected and a gum abscess may develop. The pain is continuous, severe and throbbing, with tenderness of the gum and some swelling. The tooth may become loose

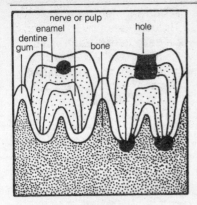

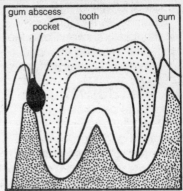

and tender to bite on. A swelling of the face on the affected side may develop.

How can toothache be prevented?

The important thing is to clean your teeth regularly so that all plaque is removed. A good diet and fluoride toothpaste, and tablets for growing children, are also important. (See whole section on *Dental Health*.)

What is the treatment?

Take painkillers such as aspirin or paracetamol, 2 tablets every 4 hours as necessary. Treat the cause.

If there is a hole:
- Rinse mouth vigorously with warm salt water (1 teaspoon of salt to 1 glass of water).
- Clean the hole with a toothbrush or toothpick.
- Fill with cotton wool soaked in oil of cloves *or* with a paste made up of zinc oxide

powder mixed with 2 or 3 drops of oil of cloves to make a temporary filling.
- Go to see a dentist as soon as possible.

If there is any swelling and you think you may have an abscess:
- Go to see a dentist as soon as possible.
- If a dentist is not available you should take a 5-day course of antibiotics such as penicillin 250mg 6-hourly (see *Common Drugs*, section 8, for alternatives).
- Rinse out your mouth frequently with hot salt water and take painkillers as necessary while you arrange to see a dentist.

For children with milk-teeth:
- Because the roots are quite shallow an abscess is likely to 'burst' through the gum having formed a gum boil. When it bursts, the pain and

swelling will quickly subside, but the child should still be seen by a dentist and may still require a course of antibiotics.

DEPRESSION

All of us experience days when we feel 'down': everything seems to go wrong, we feel close to tears or very irritable, and there seems to be a black cloud hanging over everything. It is a normal human reaction and the causes are numerous: tiredness and overwork, lack of sleep, lack of feeling appreciated, loneliness, bereavement, chronic ill health, pre-menstrual tension, a 40th birthday (or 30th, or 60th! depending on where you are!) and so on. For most of us the feelings last for a few days and when we've caught up with our sleep, had a break, or got over the problem, we find our mood has changed and we feel back to normal again.

For a small number of people these feelings persist, leading to a permanent feeling of depression. When this happens it is best *not* to try to ignore it; something has gone wrong with your chemistry. You need help.

Symptoms

The symptoms and signs of an impending or established depression are, among others:

● Constant feeling of tiredness.

● Constant feeling of 'black cloud' over you.

● Feelings of tension which are generally there all the time, or if not, then easily triggered off into irritability or over-reaction.

● Tendency to weepiness.

● Wanting to hide away, or, for some, an inability to be alone for fear your feelings might overcome you.

● Disinterest in life, your work, or the people around you: a feeling of distance from everyone.

● Increasing sense of failure or guilt, especially an inappropriate guilt.

● Inability to pray, or feeling you are not 'getting through' when you pray.

● Thoughts going around and around the same circle; sometimes the idea of suicide becomes attractive.

● Difficulty in getting off to sleep, or disturbed sleep, sometimes with vivid, disturbing dreams.

● Disinterest in food, or an excessive interest, that becomes comfort eating.

● Disinterest in appearance.

● Various physical symptoms such as abdominal pains, back-ache, headaches, palpitations, weight loss (or gain).

If you, or someone you know, is developing some of these symptoms, then you do need to see a counsellor or a doctor.

NOTE

If you, or someone you are helping, is feeling suicidal then it is *very* important to ask a doctor for help. Don't ignore this.

What is the treatment?

Talk things through with someone to try to find the underlying cause. If the cause is physical, it may have a straightforward solution. Sometimes the causes are complex and rooted in the past. Sometimes there are spiritual elements. Christians and religious people may have a particular problem here. There is often a temptation to spiritualize the whole thing and blame it on your spiritual state, God's anger or the attack of the devil. Certainly Christians believe the devil can use your depression to make you feel guilty (he is called the Accuser in the Bible). But the guilt will be inappropriate, overwhelming and not relieved by a sense of forgiveness. This is part of the depression — and it is the depression, not the guilt, that needs acknowledgment and treatment.

Medication is sometimes needed and the need is not a sign of defeat or weakness. Biochemical changes do take place in the nervous system during depression and to correct these changes it is sometimes essential to take anti-depressants.

NOTE

Some anti-depressants are taken at night as they cause drowsiness which, as a side effect, also help with disturbed sleep. They need to be taken regularly, probably for several months, to have a long-lasting effect. They must not be stopped suddenly as this can cause a severe relapse: 'coming off' them should be done gradually under medical supervision. Taking the occasional anti-depressant will do nothing for you at all, except possibly tranquillize you temporarily. Tranquillizers are sometimes given to deal with associated anxiety or tension; these can be used intermittently when you feel particularly tense, or if you have difficulty with sleeping. Drugs are very effective, but they are not sufficient in themselves to sort out depression. The underlying cause must also be dealt with.

DIABETES MELLITUS

What is it?
Diabetes is a disorder caused by under-activity of the pancreas, the organ which secretes the hormone 'insulin'. Normally, when people eat carbohydrates, such as bread, sugar or potatoes, they are turned into glucose and passed into the bloodstream. With the help of insulin, the glucose is used by the body to provide heat and energy. Without insulin, the muscles are unable to use the glucose and the level of sugar in the person's blood rises.

What is the cause?
The real cause is not known, but some people are disposed by heredity to develop diabetes, particularly if they persistently over-eat or are overweight. Sometimes diabetes may start after an infection, operation, pregnancy or emotional upheaval.

What are the symptoms?
An unquenchable thirst, and passing frequent, large amounts of urine. There may also be a loss of weight, tiredness, and recurrent skin or vaginal infections. If you have these symptoms you should see a doctor, who will do urine and blood tests.

What is the treatment?
If it is discovered that you have diabetes, you will be taught to regulate your diet to one with high fibre and low fat and to administer your own insulin. In older people, diet and tablets only may be necessary. It is **vitally important** that you adhere to your diet and insulin doses, have regular eye and general check-ups each year, and that you do not forget to take the insulin with you when you travel. It is perfectly possible for a diabetic to live a normal life, but if you develop any infections, especially of skin or urine, you will need antibiotic treatment as soon as possible, and should see a doctor quickly.

DIARRHOEA
The most important rule of all in diarrhoea is to replace the fluid that the body loses. Fluids should not be restricted because this leads to dehydration: the diarrhoea eventually stops because the gut is 'drying out' with the patient.

What is it?
Diarrhoea is usually experienced as frequent loose watery stools, sometimes accompanied by a low fever, nausea and colicky central or left-sided stomach pain.

Treatment in adults
- Stop eating solids for 24 hours.
- Increase your fluid intake by drinking weak tea, clear soups, weak squashes or diluted fruit juices (which contain potassium salts). These help to replace lost sugar and salt. Have a drink after every bowel movement. If you are vomiting, keep taking sips every few minutes instead of larger volumes every few hours.
- As the diarrhoea improves, start eating energy-giving foods such as boiled rice, soup, bread and toast, biscuits and ripe bananas (which contain potassium and a binding agent called pectin). Potatoes, yoghurt, and citrus fruits are also good (the latter provide potassium) and you should gradually resume a normal diet by about the third day. Tablets or kaolin mixture can be taken to relieve the symptoms, but sometimes only prolong general recovery.

Treatment in children
Dehydration can occur very rapidly in children and so the basic rule of replacing fluids lost is even more important. The thirst mechanism can go wrong; the child often resists feeding or drinks. This can be a real problem, and has to be overcome with patience and perseverance. Signs of dehydration are:
- Dry tongue and mouth.
- Sunken eyes.
- Skin that has lost its elasticity (does not flatten out at once when pinched up).
- Increased drowsiness.
- Sunken fontanelle (in babies).
- If severe, often no thirst.
- Scanty or no urine.

Follow the instructions to make up the oral rehydration solution (see page 104). Accurate measurements are important where babies are concerned: make sure you use the 5ml plastic teaspoon the chemists stock if possible. If the child won't drink, the solution must be spoon-fed to the child, giving 2 or 3 spoonfuls every 5 to 10 minutes until the diarrhoea and vomiting begins to stop. Sometimes a child will suck on an ice-cube or an ice lolly even if he refuses everything else: this is fine.

Oral rehydration solution

1 litre water
8×5ml teaspoon/20gm sugar or glucose
1 5ml teaspoon salt/7gm for adults
½ 5ml teaspoon salt/3.5gm for children
¼ 5ml teaspoon bicarbonate of soda or sodium citrate/2.5gm

Use the plastic 5ml teaspoon the chemists stock to give you accurate measurements. Mix the ingredients together thoroughly and drink a glassful after every bowel movement. If you are vomiting, take sips every 10–15 minutes instead of drinking it in one go: the stomach is less likely to reject it if you 'drip' it in.

Powders in sachets, such as Oralyte, can also be bought and used instead; these give you very accurately measured amounts of salts and glucose, but are expensive.

Alternative rehydration solution

Rice water has been used effectively in India, Thailand and elsewhere to treat diarrhoea. There is something in the starch of rice and rice water that 'binds' or inhibits the diarrhoea; it also provides some of the nutritional elements that are needed. Make it up as follows:

1oz/28gm rice to 1 pint/20 fluid oz water
2 teaspoons of sugar and a small pinch of salt

Wash the rice thoroughly, add the other ingredients, flavouring with lemon rind if wished, then bring to the boil and simmer for half an hour with the lid on. The liquid should then be drained off and used to feed the child initially; the rice porridge left can be saved for later and given when food is being introduced.

Treatment in babies

Continue to breast-feed while giving the extra rehydration fluid after every bowel movement or vomit. A bottle-fed baby should receive only the rehydration fluid for 24 hours, then gradually have milk re-introduced over the next 3 or 4 days. (This is done by giving quarter-strength milk on the first day, half-strength the next, three-quarter on the third and full strength on the fourth day.)

Re-introduction of food in the older baby or toddler

Rice porridge can be used, giving small frequent portions

throughout the day, rather than 1 or 2 larger meals which will probably be refused anyway. Other good foods to start with are mashed banana, fingers of toast, or biscuits. Later, mashed potatoes, rice pudding or tinned baby foods can be given (gradually returning to a normal diet over 2 or 3 days).

NOTE

Small children often get diarrhoea and vomiting with an ear or throat infection, and if they have a temperature or appear to be in pain, and the diarrhoea continues for more than 36 to 48 hours, they should be examined by a doctor in case antibiotics are needed.

DYSLEXIA

What is it?

This is a condition in which someone who has normal vision finds it difficult to interpret written language, and therefore finds it difficult to read. It often occurs in people of normal or above average intelligence, and it is more common in boys than in girls.

Dyslexic children are right- or left-handed, or ambidextrous, and are often good at subjects other than reading. In the early stages of learning, any child may transpose letters or words, or read words backwards, such as 'was' for 'saw', but this does not normally persist after the first few years. Dyslexic children may be good at memorizing so that they appear to be reading when in reality they are responding to a certain picture with the memorized words. They may find it difficult to learn correct spelling, and may not be able to recognize mistakes.

As they progress through school, frustration and the feeling of being misunderstood by teachers and their peers may cause behaviour problems. They often have difficulty in concentrating because their immediate memory span may be very short.

What can be done about it?

First, recognize that there is a real problem and be aware of the frustration and perhaps alienation or inferiority the child may be feeling.

Some teachers have special training in teaching dyslexic children, but the diagnosis has first to be made correctly. Special clinics exist for this purpose in some countries. Twenty per cent of children with dyslexia can be helped by wearing special glasses that block the vision in one eye. Specialists can sort out who these children are.

Seek advice from teachers or a doctor if you suspect your child may have this problem.

The sooner it is recognized, the sooner the child can be helped.

EAR PROBLEMS

For further information on ear problems in children, see also section 5.4.

Common problems in adults are pain in or around the ear, deafness, inflammation of the external ear canal (otitis externa) and wax.

Pain

It is unusual for an adult to get the sort of earache that children have, which is caused by a middle ear infection. Causes of pain around the ear *could* be due to an infection, but are more likely to be due to problems with the teeth; the joint between the upper and lower jaws; problems with the gland in front of and below each ear (the parotid gland), such as mumps; or impacted wax (usually associated with deafness).

Sometimes travelling in unpressurized (or badly pressurized) aircraft can cause severe pain due to the pressure difference between the environment and the inner ear. Swallowing, yawning, chewing or sucking sweets will help to equalize the pressures. If the pain persists for some days after the journey then it would be wise to have the ear checked by a doctor.

Deafness

This has many causes. The first thing to check for is wax: if there is impacted wax in the ear this will need softening with olive oil or other similar agent (1–2 drops 3 times per day for 3–4 days) and then will have to be syringed out by a nurse or doctor. For those under age 50, persistent deafness should be checked by an ear, nose and throat specialist if wax is not the cause. For those over 50, check again for wax. With age, the movements at the joints between the small bones (ossicles) in the inner ear become less accurate, leading to certain sound vibrations being less clearly transmitted. Certain tones cannot be heard: this usually leads to difficulty in distinguishing individual voices in a crowded room, or missing parts of words or sentences.

There are other causes of deafness too, of course. Hearing aids may help, but the nature and cause of the deafness should be established first so that the best hearing aid for the particular disability may be fitted.

Otitis externa

This is an inflammation of the lining of the external canal of the ear. It may be caused by trauma (such as trying to 'clean' the ear with a cotton bud), by an infection, or by eczema.

- Trauma
  Bleeding, discharge and
  infection may result. A
  couple of drops of TCP in
  the same amount of water
  may help, or Savlon cream,
  but do not use cotton buds
  to apply it. If there is
  persisting pain and
  bleeding, or if you have
  become deaf, see a doctor.
- Infection
  Antibiotic ear drops may be
  needed, but diluted TCP or
  Savlon cream may be
  sufficient. If discharge
  develops and persists, see
  a doctor.
- Eczema
  This tends to be a recurrent
  problem and the doctor may
  prescribe steroid ear drops
  to be used from time to
  time.

ECZEMA

See *Skin problems*.

EPILEPSY

See also *Convulsions* earlier in
this section and *Febrile
convulsions*, section 5.4.

What is epilepsy?

This has become a blanket
term often used wrongly to
refer to any fit. Convulsions
can be caused by many
factors: a high temperature in
a small child; scarring of the
brain tissue after a birth injury
or a head injury in later life;
and a variety of illnesses.

A convulsion occurs when
there is a sudden discharge of
'electrical' impulses through
the brain, sometimes
generalized, but sometimes
from a focus such as a scar.
The discharge of impulses can
be triggered by high
temperatures, emotional
factors, or the flickering lights
of a television.

A diagnosis of epilepsy is
made when someone has had
several convulsions and
investigations do not reveal an
on-going illness. Usually
investigations will include an
electrical brainwave recording,
known as an EEG, which will
show if there is an abnormal
pattern or a focus of some sort.

Treatment

This depends on the cause
and frequency of the attacks.
In epilepsy, the attacks are
controlled and may be stopped
altogether by regular
medication. The dosage will
need to be adjusted from time
to time and regular blood tests
(6–12 monthly) may be
advised to monitor the dose.

Long-term effects

Many people with epilepsy live
and work perfectly normally.
There has, in the past, been
quite a stigma attached to 'the
epileptic', but this is only
through fear and ignorance.
The disease can usually be
well controlled. There is a small

number of people in whom the control turns out to be a problem. These people are not normally allowed to drive and are advised not to swim. Usually driving licences will not be issued to those who have had a fit within 2 years: this is for their own as well as other people's safety.

EYE PROBLEMS

See also section 5.4 for *Conjunctivitis*, *Squint* and *Short-sightedness* in children.

'BLACK EYE'

This is really a blue or purple discolouration of the eyelids with swelling, as a result of a blow to the eye. It will take 2–3 weeks to clear completely, like any bruise, becoming yellow and gradually fading.

Apply a cold compress as soon as possible.
NOTE
A black eye from a blow to any *other* part of the head will need to be followed up by a skull X-ray in case a fracture has occurred.

CONJUNCTIVITIS

or 'Pink eye'
This is an inflammation of the lining of the eye caused by a virus or bacterium, and is accompanied by burning pain or a gritty feeling, and a clear or sticky yellow discharge.

Pink, inflamed eyes can also be the result of smoke, dust, allergies and irritants rubbed in by your hand. There is profuse watering of the eyes, but no yellow discharge or stickiness.

For bacterial or viral infections, treat with antibiotic ointment, or drops such as Chloramphenicol, Tetracycline or Sulphacetamide, inside the lower lid 2–4 times a day. See also *Common drugs*, section 8. Borax eye drops are mildly antiseptic and may be helpful. For allergic conditions, try the 'decongestant' eye drops available, such as Murine or Otrovine-Antistin. If the discomfort is caused by an irritant wash out with large amounts of cool or tepid water.
NOTE
If there is no improvement in 36–48 hours, or if there is any blurring of vision, or a misty film developing (apart from that caused by the ointment) seek medical advice as soon as possible. Eye drops and ointments should be discarded 4–6 weeks after opening the container.

CONTACT LENSES

In the heat and dust of many tropical countries, these can cause irritation. Take a spare pair of glasses with you and be especially scrupulous about the care of your lenses. Make sure you have access to a good supply of cleaning fluid. If you develop soreness or conjunctivitis, do not wear the contact lenses until your eyes are back to normal again.

EYE INJURIES

These commonly occur when a small piece of glass, metal, wood or dust flies into the eye. The object may lodge under the eyelids, causing irritation, watering of the eye and redness. The object may also become embedded in the surface of the eye leading to serious complications.

If the object is embedded, **do not attempt to remove it**. Cover the eye with a clean dressing pad and bandage gently, but firmly enough to stop the eye blinking. Go to the nearest doctor or casualty department of a hospital to have it removed as soon as possible. If you have to wait several hours (or longer) flush or bathe the eye as for conjunctivitis every 1-2 hours; if you have antibiotic eye drops or ointment, apply after each bathing. The dangers are infection and scarring, which might permanently affect your eyesight.

If the object is not embedded, flush the eye with large amounts of tepid or cold boiled water. This may wash out the object. If this does not work, turn the eyelids outwards and remove the object with a 'cotton bud' or the edge of a clean handkerchief. (Get someone else to do this for you, or look in the mirror.) Once the object is removed, treat the eye as for conjunctivitis for 2-3 days.

LONG AND SHORT SIGHT

These are caused by alterations in the shape of the eye. The focus changes to a point further away (hypermetropia) or nearer (myopia). The problem with focusing can be corrected with glasses or contact lenses.

READING

A properly trained optician will advise you if you need glasses, and can often give advice about the necessity or otherwise of seeing a doctor about any difficulties you may be having.

'RED EYE'

A bright red localized area just under the lining of the eye (conjunctiva), usually in the inner or outer triangle of the white part of the eye, is the result of a small blood-vessel bursting. This is quite harmless and usually painless, though there may be some irritation from the swelling. It is the result of straining or coughing.

No treatment is necessary. An eye bath of Optrex or dilute salt solution may be soothing. It clears up over a few days as the blood becomes re-absorbed.

NOTE
If the *whole* white of the eye is

red, with pain, but no discharge or stickiness, seek medical advice urgently. Check for deterioration of vision: shut the good eye and see if there is any change in the clarity of vision. If your vision is not as clear as usual in that eye seek **urgent** medical advice.

STYE

A stye is an infection in the base of an eyelash, causing the development of a boil.

Treat with hot compresses, by wrapping a clean piece of cloth around a wooden spoon, dipping it in warm to hot boiled water (check it is not too hot; it should not burn), squeezing out gently and applying to the affected eye. A cloth used alone in the same way would also be effective. Reapply when the compress has become cold. This will help to bring the boil to a head.

The whole thing may be prevented from developing further by gently pulling out the eyelash with a pair of tweezers. This may lead to discharge of the pus. **Do not squeeze the stye**.

Antibiotic ointment rubbed gently into the eyelid at the base of the eyelashes 2 or 3 times daily for a few days may help.

TRACHOMA

This is a chronic bacterial infection very common in the tropics. The symptoms are similar to those of conjunctivitis. It can cause permanent scarring or long-term eye problems.

FAINTING

What is it?

This is a sudden loss of consciousness caused by a fall in blood pressure. Just before the faint occurs there is usually a feeling of light-headedness, with a sense of everything going dark (a 'black-out') and perhaps a cold sweat and feeling of fear or panic.

It is often the result of pain, blood loss or an emotional shock, but it may also occur in someone who is anaemic, or who hasn't been eating regularly. Some people experience the light-headedness and feeling of darkness if they get up suddenly from sitting or lying down: this is because the blood pressure hasn't had time to adjust itself to the new position.

Treatment

● If you feel faint, lie down flat with your legs raised above the level of your head. If you cannot lie flat, put your head down between your knees and breathe quietly and deeply.

● If someone else has fainted, loosen any tight clothing and raise the legs up above head level by putting a pillow or box under them. This will usually encourage a quick recovery but the person should stay resting quietly in this position for a while.

NOTE

If the recovery does not occur within 30 seconds or 1 minute of raising the legs, get urgent medical help. Check pulse and breathing, and if necessary start mouth-to-mouth resuscitation and heart massage while awaiting medical help. (See *First aid at the roadside*, section 2.4.)

FEVER

What is it?

A normal body temperature is below 37°C/98.4°F. A fever is a rise in this temperature, usually as a result of infection. A small rise is acceptable as it indicates that the body defences are working to heal the body. Above certain levels it can cause problems, however. If possible, the cause should be discovered and treated specifically, but sometimes this is difficult. Virus infections, for example, do not respond to antibiotics, so only the symptoms of viral illnesses such as influenza can be treated. However, bacterial infections, such as tonsillitis, middle-ear infections, skin infections which cause a fever, should be treated with antibiotics, as well as the measures for controlling the fever. Malaria should of course be treated with anti-malarials (see *Malaria*, section 6).

To control the temperature: *in adults*

There is no danger until the temperature rises above 40°C/104°F, but the general aches and pains in muscles, back and head caused by the fever can be relieved to some extent by:

● 2 aspirin or paracetamol given every 4 hours.
● Plenty of cold drinks — a constant supply, as fluid is lost in sweating.
● Placing the person in a slight breeze of fresh air or a draught from a fan, with a light covering only.

If the temperature rises above 40°C/104°F:

● Give a cool bath or cool shower but do not dry: allow the water evaporation to cool down the body.

OR

● Wet the person all over and leave to dry in the air if unable to get up; keep wetting and allow to dry until temperature comes down.

To control the temperature: *in children*

A temperature above 39°C/102°F should be brought down as soon as possible, especially in babies and children under 5 as there is a risk of a febrile convulsion. (See also *Febrile convulsions*, section 5.4.)

● Strip the child and wet him *all over* with tepid water. Allow the air to dry the body naturally: the evaporation brings the temperature down. This is helped by a cool breeze or draught. Repeat the wetting and air-drying until the temperature comes down. The child can also be repeatedly immersed in a tepid bath and lifted out to dry in the air until the temperature comes down.

This is not a very pleasant process, but the child will feel *very* much better once the temperature is down. It will not cause the child to 'catch pneumonia'.

● Give aspirin or paracetamol in the appropriate dosage, every 4 hours, if necessary. This will help to keep the temperature down for 3–4 hours, but you may have to repeat the tepid sponging when the effect wears off.

Crush tablets up in a spoon with honey, jam or suitable alternative to make them more pleasant to take.

FIBROSITIS
(Fibromyositis)

What is it?

This is a general term applied to pain, and sometimes stiffness, felt in muscles, joints and the associated fibrous tissues where there is probably some inflammation. Another term loosely applied to similar pain is *Rheumatism*.

What causes it?

It is sometimes caused by trauma, exposure to cold and damp, and occasionally by virus or other infections. The pain and stiffness may be felt more severely if you are under stress or particularly tired.

What are the symptoms?

The pain may come on suddenly or gradually, and may be aggravated by movement. There may be a particularly tender spot or nodule. There is sometimes muscle spasm around the area.

As all these symptoms have other causes too, consult a doctor if it persists for more than a week or two, or if it rapidly becomes worse.

How should it be treated?

● Rest the affected part.
● Apply a hot-water bottle or similar to the area several times a day, or whenever you are sitting down.

- Massage the muscle or area gently several times a day.
- Take aspirin, 2 tablets 3 or 4 times a day for a week or so, to kill the pain and reduce inflammation.
- If the pain persists and is very severe, a doctor may inject the tender spot with a steroid preparation.

FOOD ALLERGY

There has been a great deal of interest and research into this in recent years. There are still many differences of opinion about the subject in medical circles, and many immunologists would argue that there is no such thing as a 'food allergy', but that it is more a case of individuals being particularly sensitive to specific substances. However, the term 'food allergy' is in general use for such sensitivities.

What is it?

It is an abnormal response to a food, or substances used in foods, such as colourings and other additives. It may develop as soon as a particular food is introduced in infancy, or it may develop later, at any time in life. Any food or drink may cause it, but some do so more frequently than others.

What are the symptoms?

There are a whole host of these, among them:

- Eczema.
- Asthma or wheezing.
- Hay fever, or a runny nose and watering eyes.
- Persistent coughs.
- Migraines, or severe headaches.
- 'Glue ears' in children, caused by the production of a sticky fluid that does not drain away from the middle ear.
- Behaviour problems or sudden mood changes, such as hyperactivity in some children who rush about, unable to sit still at all, or who have sudden temper tantrums or are unable to concentrate, often with a sudden exhaustion at the end of such a period of hyperactivity; or in adults, *some* sudden and inexplicable mood changes.

How can it be diagnosed?

- Parents should take note of the above symptoms in children and note the foods eaten in the previous 12–24 hours or so; or the sudden absence of certain foods or drinks of which the child may have eaten or drunk a lot previously. Occasionally, symptoms may be due to withdrawal of substances to which the person has become 'addicted'. Keep a record for a few weeks or months.
- Take the record and the

child to see a doctor to discuss your observations.

● In some centres it is possible to test for food allergies directly, but there are not many such centres as yet.

How can it be treated?

● You may be advised to avoid certain foods for a particular period of time, perhaps a month or longer, depending on the problem. This means cutting it out altogether from the diet. If it is believed that cow's milk is responsible, for example, all foods which may contain cow's milk, such as cakes, ice-cream, biscuits, and puddings, must be avoided. If it is food colouring, it will be necessary to read all food labels carefully and avoid *all* foods or medicines which have this colouring.

● After the specific period of avoidance, a small amount of the substance should be introduced and the effects observed over the next few days. Gradually increase the amount eaten. If symptoms recur, you should return to avoidance of the substance for perhaps 3–6 months. It may be possible, then, to re-introduce it gradually again as the sensitivity may have been corrected. Some people remain sensitive to the food all their lives.

Severe or complicated cases

Sometimes people are sensitive to several substances, or they may not develop symptoms until there is a certain level or combination of all these substances in the body. This takes a much more complicated process to sort out than the one described, and expert guidance on elimination and rotation diets is needed.

FLAT FEET

What are they?

All feet should have a natural arch along the inner border of the foot to give it a 'spring' when walking. When this arch becomes lax and drops or flattens out, the foot is said to become 'flat'. Toddlers often look as though they have flat feet, usually because the arch hasn't developed completely as yet; there is no need to take corrective action, except to ensure that the child has good strong shoes to protect and support the feet.

What are the symptoms?

There may be pain in the foot, especially in the arch region, but also elsewhere, sometimes even felt in the ankles, knees, hips or lower back, because of the altered weight-bearing on these joints.

What can be done about them?

- Wear good supportive shoes.
- Do foot exercises by picking up marbles with your toes, or standing on tip-toe, or rising up and down on tip-toe 20 times several times a day.
- Place arch supports, such as those made out of sponge in your shoes.
- Take aspirin, 2 tablets, 4-hourly and rest, if the pain is severe.
- See a doctor for an examination if the pain persists or is very severe.

GALL BLADDER PROBLEMS

STONES

The pain from gall stones is severe and sudden, and occurs on the right side of the upper abdomen, often radiating round to the back.

The gall bladder stores bile, which helps the digestion of fats. A fatty meal causes it to contract to 'send' the bile out into the gut. Gall stones may block the exit, or get stuck in the duct, and the pain is caused by the gall bladder or duct contracting hard to overcome the blockage. Avoid rich or fatty foods and see a doctor as soon as possible.

How can it be treated?

- Sometimes by tablets.
- Usually by operation to remove the gall stones.

CHOLECYSTITIS

This is an inflammation or infection of the gall bladder. It can happen with or without gall stones. The pain is more constant in the upper right half of the abdomen, but is particularly severe after a fatty meal, and may cause vomiting.

How should it be treated?

- Avoid rich and fatty foods.
- Sometimes doctors prescribe antibiotics.
- Rest and anti-nausea tablets such as Stemetil or Maxolon may help to settle the symptoms.

GERMAN MEASLES (Rubella)

See also *Immunization*, section 4.1.

What is it?

This is a mild viral infection causing a pink rash on the face, body and limbs, lasting 2–3 days. If rubella occurs in pregnancy, especially in the first 3 months, it can cause damage to the unborn child. Girls should be immunized against rubella before puberty to prevent this risk.

What is the treatment?

If you suspect that you have

rubella, stay away from women of child-bearing age, and treat your illness as you would a mild fever. There are no antibiotics for this illness.
NOTE
If you are pregnant and think you have had contact with rubella see a doctor: some hospitals can do a blood test to see if you are already immune and gamma-globulin can be given to protect you and the baby if you are not.

GLANDULAR FEVER

What is it?
This is a viral illness (also known as infectious mononucleosis) to which young adults are particularly prone. The symptoms are a very sore throat, enlargement and tenderness of the glands, especially those in the neck, and fever with weakness, lethargy and loss of appetite. A rash may appear on the face and body. Diagnosis can only be made by specific blood tests.

What is the treatment?
Antibiotics are not effective, and complete recovery may take several weeks or months.
● The person should stay in bed while the fever is present, eat a simple diet, avoid alcohol and take plenty of rest until normal

health is restored.
● Relapses of the illness may occur if there is a return to normal activity too quickly.
● Some people become quite depressed, as with hepatitis, but this passes with full recovery.

GONORRHOEA
See *Sexually transmitted diseases*.

GOUT
See *Joint pains*.

HEADACHES
Almost everyone suffers from headaches from time to time. There are a large number of causes, and if you have a tendency to headaches it is as well to learn to recognize under what circumstances you are likely to develop one and to take avoiding action if possible!
   The most common types of headache are tension and migraine. There is a tendency to call any severe headache a migraine, but not all severe headaches are migraine, and not all attacks of migraine cause headaches!

TENSION HEADACHES

What are they?
Tension headaches are extremely common. They are usually described in terms

such as 'a tight band round the head', or 'the top of my head feels as though it's about to burst'. There is often a pain above or around one or both eyes, or focused in one temple, or just a general dull ache over the whole of the top of the head.

Causes

There are many causes: tension, tiredness, straining to read in poor light, not having eaten for hours, or not drinking enough fluid on a hot day, for example. Anxiety, anger, or just being constantly under pressure causes muscle tensions, especially in the muscles around the neck and shoulders. Several of these are attached to the base of the skull and the scalp which is loose over the top of the head, attached above the eyes and at the base of the skull. When the muscles are tense, the scalp is under constant tension and this is what ends up feeling like a headache.

What is the treatment?

- Try to correct the cause of the tension; eat or drink something; lie down if you can.
- Take aspirin or paracetamol, 2 tablets every 4–6 hours.
- Learn muscle relaxation techniques if you are prone to tension headaches.

MIGRAINE HEADACHES

What are they?

Migraine headaches are quite different although they can also be triggered by tension — or the release of tension, as at a weekend or the beginning of a holiday. They are caused by the dilation of blood-vessels over the surface of the head. This reaction can be triggered off by a variety of foods such as chocolate, cheese, coffee, marmite and red wine. It can also be triggered by flashing lights, anger, tension and so on. Those with a tendency to migraines should note what they have eaten in the 24 hours before the attack and learn to avoid their 'trigger factor'.

A typical attack

- May start with nausea, flashing or flickering kaleidoscope light formations, different for everyone.
- Increasingly severe headache, perhaps on one side of the head only.
- Increasing dislike of light, increasing nausea, perhaps vomiting.
- Severe headache with nausea and vomiting persisting for 36 hours or more.
- Some people experience bizarre 'nerve' symptoms such as pins and needles, or numbness in the hand.

● Many people see flickering or flashing lights before the headache starts; others find that 'chunks' seem to have disappeared out of words or letters when they try to read.

For some, vomiting will relieve the headache and the recovery will start once they are able to go to sleep, so cutting short the attack.

Treatment
● Avoid trigger factors.
● At the *first* sign of attack (nausea or flashing lights, for example) take an anti-emetic such as Maxolon (metoclopramide) or Stemetil and go and lie down quietly if possible. A 5mg dose of Diazepam or other tranquillizers may be very helpful too.
● After 20–30 minutes, take 2–3 *soluble* aspirin or paracetamol. The Maxolon will have settled your stomach so that the aspirin can be absorbed properly and quickly.

Stay resting, if possible sleeping, for an hour or so. This treatment will often successfully abort an attack and if you catch the attack early enough, it may be all that is needed.

For some, however, this is not enough. Stronger medication will be needed, such as Ergotamine, which will counteract the dilation of the blood vessels. This and stronger pain-killers should only be used on the advice of your doctor, as excessive use of Ergotamine can in itself cause migraine-type headaches.

Other useful treatments include Migraleve, Soluble Migravess, Migril, all of which contain an anti-emetic and pain-killer in one tablet.

MISCELLANEOUS HEADACHES
Persistent severe headaches that do not fall into either of the above categories, or that do not respond to the suggested measures, should be discussed with a doctor when possible. Influenza and other febrile illnesses such as malaria, of course, cause severe headaches sometimes.

HEART ATTACK

What is it?
This occurs when the blood supply to a part of the heart muscle is suddenly cut off. The result depends on how much of the heart muscle is affected. It is usually accompanied by sudden, severe chest pain.

Causes
It may happen as a result of a blood clot blocking the passage through a blood-vessel: this is known as a coronary thrombosis. It may be

the result of a 'plaque' of fatty material (such as cholesterol) building up on the wall of the blood-vessel and blocking it: this is called atherosclerosis. People who have 'furred up' blood-vessels generally, or who have high blood pressure, or who may have had episodes of angina (see *Angina*, earlier in this section) previously, are more likely to have heart attacks. It is possible to have one with no previous history of angina or any other problem. It is very rare for anyone below the age of 40 to have any heart problems of this sort. Smoking increases the risk of having heart attacks.

How can heart attacks be prevented?

- Stop smoking: even if you have smoked for years, you are less likely to have a heart attack if you stop now.
- Eat a sensible diet, and bring up your children to do the same. Keep it low in cholesterol, fat and salt and high in fibre.
- Take regular and moderate amounts of exercise. If you have not been exercising for years, take care to start slowly and build up in easy stages: go for short frequent walks, lengthen them over a period of weeks, then start jogging or doing other exercises as you become fitter.

What does a heart attack feel like?

Some or all of the following may be felt:

- Sudden severe pain across the chest, starting, or felt mostly, on the left side: it may be described as a gripping pain or like a vice around the chest.
- Pain may spread up into the neck or go down into the left arm.
- A feeling of panic.
- A choking sensation and perhaps difficulty in breathing.

The person will be in obvious pain, perhaps be panicking and will usually be pale and sweating, sometimes having difficulty in breathing.

What to do

If someone seems to be having a heart attack, don't waste time: send for a doctor or an ambulance at once.

- If the person is able to tell you, find out where the pain is so that you can tell the doctor when he asks you.
- Loosen any tight clothing around the neck to help with breathing.
- Make the person as comfortable as possible.
- If the person carries pills or a spray for angina, find them and give him a dose at once while waiting for the ambulance or doctor. The usual tablets are called glyceryl trinitrate. One is

placed under the tongue where it dissolves and works within 1–2 minutes. The spray is a similar substance: this is sprayed onto the tongue and works even more quickly.

- If you have no pills or spray, a small glass of brandy may help.

If the patient suddenly becomes unconscious, and stops breathing, **start mouth-to-mouth resuscitation and cardiac massage** at once, and continue until the doctor or ambulance arrives. (See *First aid*, section 2.3.)

After a heart attack
When you have recovered from a heart attack:

- Get back to as normal a life as possible, but work towards it gradually over a period of about 6 or more weeks.
- Take regular exercise, but in the first couple of months avoid sudden vigorous bursts of energy: it is unwise to play vigorous games or have sexual intercourse. Gradually increase the amount and vigour of your exertions over several weeks.
- Don't smoke.
- Drink alcohol only in moderation, if at all.
- Maintain a low cholesterol and low salt diet.
- Have your blood pressure checked regularly, that is,

every 3–6 months, according to your doctor's advice.
- Take whatever medication your doctor or specialist has advised.

HERNIA

What is it?
A hernia is a protrusion of a part of the gut through a weakness in the abdominal wall. There are several types; the common ones are discussed briefly here.

UMBILICAL
This occurs in some babies. It usually causes no problem: the gut pushes out through a finger-sized area of weakness under the navel when the baby cries or strains, and goes back easily when the baby is at rest, or if pushed in.

The weakness usually closes up as the baby grows, and no treatment is necessary unless the hernia cannot be pushed back into the abdominal cavity (or 'reduced').

INGUINAL — in young boys
This type may occur if the canal in the groin through which the testes descend into the scrotum during development — the inguinal canal — does not close up properly.

A simple operation to close up the weakness is usually all

that is required; there is no immediate urgency.

INGUINAL — in adults

In the older person (usually male) it may occur as a result of straining or lifting. There is usually pain at the time of the 'rupture' and a bulge develops either in the groin or going down into the scrotum on the same side, following the line of the inguinal canal.

An operation may be necessary or a 'truss' may be worn, which presses against the weakness, preventing the gut from pushing out into it. If the gut gets 'stuck' in the scrotum and cannot be pushed back into the abdominal cavity, an obstruction in the intestines may result and an emergency operation would have to be done. There will be pain and swelling at the site of the hernia, with stomach cramps and vomiting.

HIATUS HERNIA

Here the stomach pushes up into the lung cavity through a weakness in the diaphragm. Common symptoms of this are a sour-tasting fluid suddenly gushing up into the mouth, known as water-brash, which happens especially on bending over or lying down; and indigestion with a burning feeling up the middle of the chest.

What is the treatment?

Losing weight, antacids (milk and tablets such as Rennies and magnesium trisilicate), sleeping on 3 – 4 pillows and avoiding tight clothing around the waist, will help a hiatus hernia. Sometimes an operation is necessary.

HERPES

See *Sexually transmitted diseases*.

HOUSEMAID'S KNEE

See *Joint pains*.

HYPERTENSION

See *Blood pressure*.

HYPERVENTILATION

What is it?

It means overbreathing: breathing too fast or too deeply. This causes the carbon dioxide in the lungs to be blown off so that the usual proportions of oxygen and carbon dioxide become unbalanced. The person literally suffers from an overdosage of oxygen.

What are the symptoms?
- Tingling in the fingers and hands, also around the mouth.
- A light-headed or 'dizzy feeling'.

- If the overbreathing continues the person may develop a type of spasm in the fingers and face called tetany where the fingers become stiffly held together, and the muscles around the mouth become stiff or go into spasm. This usually frightens the person so that he or she overbreathes even more, making the tetany worse.

What you can do

- In the early stages, try to calm the person. Get them to take steady, slow breaths, give them something to drink to break the fast breathing cycle, and try to distract their attention from the breathing.
- If this does not succeed get the person to breathe in and out of a paper bag (**not** a plastic bag) for 10 minutes or so. This will help to build up the carbon dioxide level in the lungs again and reduce the symptoms, thereby reducing the panic.

HYSTERIA

What is it?

It can mean the uncontrollable screaming, crying or similar behaviour that some people exhibit when faced with a sudden shock such as news of someone's death, or a sudden threat that causes fear.

It can also mean the much less obvious chronic problems that some people develop after a severe road-traffic accident, or other injury, where the physical healing is complete but, for example, the pain persists. See also *Hyperventilation*.

How can it be treated?

The first kind of hysterical reaction discussed can be dealt with by administering a sudden 'counter-shock' such as a sharp slap or cold water thrown over the person. Even if nothing is done the attack will usually cause exhaustion and the person will calm down.

The second kind of hysteria requires the skilled help of a psychiatrist or psychologist.

IMPETIGO

See *Skin problems*.

INDIGESTION

What is it?

This can occur after a large, greasy, spicy or hurried meal, or if you leave your stomach empty for long periods of time. The stomach produces extra acid, which gives a feeling of discomfort or burning pain in the upper abdomen, and going up the centre of the chest.

How should it be treated?

If you find this happening

persistently, you should see a doctor to determine the cause, and then take the medicine prescribed for you. Meanwhile, avoid alcohol, strong coffee, very hot drinks, smoking, spices and pepper, fizzy drinks and fatty food. Try to avoid going for long periods without a meal: have regular, fairly small meals. If you feel the pain occurring when you are hungry, drink some milk and/or take an antacid such as Aludrox, Nulacin or Rennies. If the pain occurs after a meal, an antacid may help if taken immediately after the meal. Avoid taking tablets containing aspirin, as these can irritate your stomach.

INFERTILITY

What is it?

The inability to conceive children is known as infertility. A couple will not usually be investigated until they have been trying to conceive for 18–24 months, unless there is some pressing reason, or indication that there is a health problem. It is usual for both partners to be investigated and counselled especially if advice is sought in an Infertility Clinic. Often tension and anxiety can affect the ability to conceive, and once this has been sorted out, conception will occur. Anyone who is worrying about this would be wise to discuss their worry with a doctor or someone else who can help.

What are the causes?

There are numerous causes, the following being some of the more common:

In men
● A low or inadequate production of sperm.
● A faulty production of sperm.

These problems may be caused by a blockage, or damage to the testes as a result of mumps, for example. Some boys are born with testes that have never developed and that do not produce sperm, or there may be a hormone problem.

In women
● Blockage of the Fallopian tubes.
● Ovaries that do not produce eggs regularly or at all.
● Hormone problems.

Some, but not all, of these problems can be corrected by medicines or surgery. Infertility is surprisingly common, affecting roughly 1 in every 10 couples.

INFLUENZA

What is it?

This is a highly infectious disease caused by a virus and spread by droplets from the mouths and noses of infected people.

What are the symptoms?

The start is often similar to the common cold, but other symptoms vary.

● There will always be fever and aching in back and limbs which is sometimes severe.

● There will often be a headache, sore throat and a cough, and sometimes also nausea, vomiting and some diarrhoea with abdominal pain.

The temperature normally lasts for 3–4 days and the symptoms then begin to settle.

● If you are coughing up yellow or green phlegm, you may need antibiotics.

● If you have fever, diarrhoea and abdominal pain, lasting for longer than 4–5 days, you should see a doctor, if possible.

● If the temperature does not come down *at all* with aspirin, you should see a doctor.

Malaria can cause similar symptoms, but will normally be accompanied by severe attacks of uncontrollable shivering as the temperature rises (rigors) and will be over more quickly.

What is the treatment?

● Antibiotics do not cure influenza as it is caused by a virus.

● Take aspirin or paracetamol 4-hourly.

● Stay in bed until your temperature has been normal for 1 or 2 days: this way you will recover more quickly and you will be less likely to spread the virus.

● Have a light diet and plenty to drink.

● Don't start active work until all symptoms have disappeared, as relapses of the illness, and depression, are fairly common, if you go back to work too soon.

NOTE
Influenza in children
It is advisable not to give aspirin when treating children, as there is some evidence that it may, rarely, cause a serious complication known as Reye's Disease. In this condition, the child suddenly becomes much worse, having apparently started to recover. Use paracetamol instead if something is necessary for the control of symptoms.

INGROWING TOE NAILS

This is a common problem and is caused by the nail (usually of the big toe) growing in too curved a fashion so that it digs into the skin on either side. This can be very painful, and can also cause an infection along the side of the nail.

How can they be prevented?

Cut your toe nails straight across with a v-nick centrally: this will encourage the sides to grow straight.

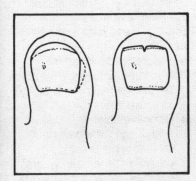

What is the treatment?

Gently lift the nail up from the sides with a cotton bud or similar. Cut down the side of the nail, if necessary, where it lifts away from the skin. (Be careful not to cut the skin.) Soak the foot in Savlon or other antiseptic mixture for 5 – 10 minutes. Using a pair of tweezers, pack the space between nail and skin with some cotton soaked in Savlon, repeating daily.

For more severe cases, antibiotics may be necessary. If there is a lot of redness and swelling with perhaps a yellow-white collection of pus at the side of the nail, take Tetracycline 250mg 4 times a day or Ampicillin 250mg 4 times a day, for 7 days (see *Common drugs*, section 8, for alternatives). The pus should be released with a needle made sterile by passing through a flame.

In recurring cases, a wedge resection may need to be done surgically.

INSOMNIA

What is it?

The term insomnia means either the inability to sleep, or disturbed sleep.

What are the causes?

The causes may be obvious and, hopefully, easy to correct: hunger, noise or light, an uncomfortable bed, a room that is too hot or too draughty, itching or pain. Some people need more sleep than others, depending on their age, work and constitution, and insomnia is often more annoying than serious.

Suggestions for dealing with it

● Anxiety or depression may

prevent you sleeping, and you would be well advised to talk over your problems and try to eliminate them.

- Avoid large meals or large quantities of drink just before bed; 'horror' films and stories of violence are also best avoided.
- Over-work and an over-stimulated mind can cause insomnia, so try to have a period of relaxation before you settle to sleep (see *Relaxation*, section 1.4).
- As a last resort, a doctor may prescribe a mild sedative (see special note) for a short while, to help you establish a healthier pattern of sleep.

NOTE

A short-acting sleeping tablet, such as Temazepam 10mg (which gives about 5-6 hours of sleep, and no hangover) may be very useful if taken for about 1 week, then intermittently, then occasionally as necessary. A mild tranquillizer may be taken in the same way for short periods. This is less dependence-inducing than the longer-acting ones such as Nitrazepam, or the barbiturates which should be avoided as they are highly addictive.

JOINT PAINS

If you develop pains in *several joints* at the same time, you should be seen by a doctor.

The pains may be the start of a viral illness such as hepatitis or influenza, and they may be accompanied by swelling and stiffness of the joints. Whatever the cause, you should rest in bed and take aspirin or paracetamol, 2 tablets every 4 hours, which will help until you can be seen by a doctor. Long-term causes of joint pains are rheumatoid arthritis or, in older people, osteo-arthritis.

Pains and swelling or stiffness in *single joints* may be due to trauma, osteo-arthritis or joint infections. Some temporary relief may be gained by resting the painful joint and applying warmth.

Some of these joint pains include:

- 'Housemaid's knee', a swollen painful knee caused by trauma (such as kneeling to scrub floors).
- 'Tennis-elbow', a swollen and/or painful elbow caused by inflammation of the capsule or the point where muscles are attached to the joint capsule, caused by vigorous, repeated movements involving the elbow, such as playing tennis.
- 'Bursitis', a swelling, with inflammation, of a bursa or 'pocket' of the lining of a joint where the 'pocket' becomes filled with fluid and pushes out from the side of the joint, causing a swelling.

● 'Gout', caused by deposits of uric acid crystals in a joint.

What is the treatment?
If you have a temperature and the joint is red, hot and swollen, see a doctor as soon as possible. Otherwise:
● Rest.
● Bandage the joint or give other support.
● Anti-inflammatory tablets such as aspirin, 2 tablets 4-hourly for several days.
See a doctor if it does not improve or keeps recurring.

LEGIONNAIRE'S DISEASE

What is it?
This is an illness caused by the organism Legionella Pneumophilia. It spreads through showers and air-conditioning systems using water which is not adequately chlorinated. The organism breeds in the moist and warm environment of a shower head or air-conditioning system and is inhaled when, for example, the shower is turned on. It causes pneumonia in the first instance; death may occur in about 10% of people, but this is usually in the elderly and those who suffer from poor health anyway.

How can it be avoided?
Run the shower for a few minutes before getting under it. Hotels and public institutions are more aware of Legionnaire's Disease, and are increasingly taking steps to reduce the problem.

What is the treatment?
For treatment, see *Pneumonia*.

LONG SIGHT
See *Eye problems*.

MENINGITIS

What is it?
It is an inflammation of the lining of the brain caused by a viral or bacterial infection. There are a number of common viruses and bacteria which can cause this, but it is not a common illness, although sometimes epidemics may occur. It can happen at any age.

What are the symptoms?
● There may be other symptoms of illness, such as a cold, or mumps, or tonsillitis.
● A severe headache, not relieved by aspirin.
● Fever.
● Pain in the head and/or back of the neck and back on bending the head forward to touch the chin to the chest, or to touch the

forehead to the knees.
- There may be vomiting.
- There may be increasing drowsiness.

If you suspect that someone has meningitis, you must call a doctor, or travel to see one as soon as possible. See section 3 for what to do on a journey to hospital.

How is it diagnosed?
- The above symptoms and findings on examination.
- By 'tapping off' some of the fluid in the spine to examine it under the microscope for changes in its usual composition, a process known as a 'lumbar puncture'.

How is it treated?
This depends on the findings of the examination and the lumbar puncture:
- If it is caused by a virus, no antibiotics are necessary, but full nursing care and treatment of the symptoms.
- If it is caused by bacteria, antibiotics are given, often by intravenous injection, or sometimes directly into the spinal canal, with full nursing care and follow-up.

How long does it take to recover?
It may be only a couple of weeks, but could take several weeks or even some months, depending on the cause and the severity.

MENTAL ILLNESS
See *Psychiatric problems*.

MIGRAINE
See *Headaches*.

NOSE BLEED

What is it?
This is usually the result of detachment of a crust in the nose, though it may occur spontaneously in women at the time of the menstrual cycle. In older people it is often associated with high blood pressure, and this should be checked. In children it is often associated with nose-picking, but there may also be an area which is inflamed and bleeds easily.

Treatment
1 Blow nose gently to remove clots.
2 Sit up and bend the head forward. Apply firm pressure to the nostrils, just below the nasal bone, with thumb and index finger, for at least 10 minutes.
3 This may be combined with ice or cold compresses applied to the side of the nose that is bleeding.
4 Allow the blood to dribble into a bowl rather than swallowing it, as you are likely to feel sick or vomit if you do.
5 If still bleeding after 30

minutes, the nose may need packing by a doctor or nurse. Continue to apply pressure just below the central bone, pressing the nostrils firmly together, until you are seen by the doctor.

PEPTIC ULCER

What is it?

It is an ulcer in the lining of the stomach or the first part of the intestines (the duodenum). It may develop quickly (acute) or slowly and persist for a long time, causing scarring (chronic).

What causes it?

The stomach normally produces enzymes and hydrochloric acid to help break down and start digesting the food. Some people produce a higher than normal amount of acid, thus causing an ulcer; others may do this in response to stress. But many other factors may be involved in the production of an ulcer, including:

● Smoking.
● Drinking alcohol.
● Taking aspirin or other drugs that irritate the lining of the stomach.
● Acute stress such as an operation, or an accident.
● Drinking very hot liquids.

What are the symptoms?

● In the early stages there may only be a discomfort in the upper middle part of the abdomen after eating, or a burning sensation there and going up the central part of the chest (see illustration, *Abdominal pain*, earlier in this section).
● Nausea is common, sometimes vomiting.
● Pain felt in the upper middle part of the abdomen, coming on up to 2 hours after eating.
● Tenderness on palpation over the same area.
● Weight loss: see a doctor if you are losing weight at a rate of 7lb or 3–4 kg in a month.

What is the treatment?

● Antacids, to neutralize the acid and 'coat' the stomach to protect the lining. (See *Common drugs*, section 8.)
● Milky drinks.
● Small, frequent meals (every 2–3 hours) to ensure the stomach is not empty for too long.
● Stop smoking, drinking alcohol and try, if possible, to reduce your stress levels. (See *Health maintenance*, section 1.3.)
● Allow hot drinks to cool before drinking them. If the above measures do not help, arrange to see a doctor, who may prescribe better antacids, or tablets that reduce the acid production and promote

healing. If necessary he may refer you to a surgeon for an X-ray or for a gastroscopy where a fine fibre optic light tube is used to look directly into the stomach and duodenum, making a diagnosis possible. Sometimes an operation is necessary.

PERITONITIS

What is it?
It is an infection and inflammation of the membrane that lines the inside of the abdomen and which surrounds the organs.

What causes it?
An escape of infected material from:
- A burst appendix or peptic ulcer.
- An infected Fallopian tube (salpingitis).
- A ruptured diverticulum which is a pocket formed when the lining of the gut becomes weakened, often as a result of chronic constipation or sometimes as a result of a typhoid illness.

What are the symptoms?
- Extreme pain in the abdomen, worsened by *any* movement, even breathing. The wall of the abdomen is held rigid to 'guard' the tissues below.
- High fever, perhaps delirium.
- Vomiting and other signs of severe illness.

What is the treatment?
Immediate admission to hospital. If you have to travel:
- Make the patient as comfortable as possible, on one side or in the recovery position, and well supported so that bumpy or rocking movements are minimized.
- Give 1 or 2 sips of water every 5–10 minutes.
- Stay with the patient throughout the journey: your presence will be re-assuring even to someone who is delirious; he may need restraining at times, and help if vomiting.
- Do *not* give any medication, even for pain.

In hospital the patient will be treated with intravenous fluids and antibiotics, and, in some cases, by operation, to 'plug' the source of infection or remove a burst appendix.

PHLEBITIS and THROMBO-PHLEBITIS

What is it?
Phlebitis is an inflammation of the veins, usually in the lower leg. Thrombosis is the formation of a blood clot in a vein. These may be associated with varicose veins, chronic

constipation, pregnancy, obesity, or just not moving the legs sufficiently such as after an operation. Those who smoke, or who are taking the contraceptive Pill, are more likely to suffer from one of these problems.

What are the symptoms of phlebitis?

- Pain and tenderness along the length of the leg, or part of it, along the line of the vein, which becomes solid and thickened.
- There may be some swelling and redness around the painful area, or swelling of the ankle on that side.

What are the symptoms of thrombophlebitis?

- Thrombophlebitis in the deep veins of the calf (a deep vein thrombosis or DVT) causes severe pain deep in the calf on walking and on pressure.
- There may be swelling and the affected calf may feel hotter than the other.
- A clot may dislodge and shoot off into the bloodstream (this is called an embolism). If it lodges in one of the arteries of the lungs it may cause a sudden cough with chest pain and difficulty with breathing. If this happens you must be examined by a doctor urgently.

How is phlebitis treated?

- Firm supportive bandage, stocking or, for example, Tubigrip.
- Keep moving the leg by walking or exercising it when sitting.
- Sit with the leg up on a low stool.
- Take aspirin, 2 tablets (300mg×2) 6-8 hourly for the anti-inflammatory effect, which will also help the pain.
- Stop taking the contraceptive Pill.

How is thrombophlebitis treated?

- Firm supportive bandage as for phlebitis.
- Stop the contraceptive Pill.
- Rest the leg and see a doctor as soon as possible: this requires anticoagulant therapy and follow-up.
- Take aspirin, 2 tablets (300mg×2) 6-8 hourly until you have seen the doctor.

PHOBIAS

What are they?

These are irrational, illogical fears about something, flying, spiders, wide-open spaces, crowds, being typical examples. People who suffer from these fears cannot overcome them by logical argument. The fear takes the form of panic attacks which produce physical symptoms such as a dry mouth, nausea, a fast heart rate and an immediate need to get away from the situation or object that triggered the reflex. It may have its origin in early childhood experiences in some cases.

How can they be dealt with?

They cannot always be overcome, but it is possible to learn how to control the panic attack and the sudden severe symptoms that occur with them. It is possible to 'unlearn' the reflex by careful training known as behavioural therapy, but this usually needs the help of a skilled counsellor or psychologist, and it often helps to be in contact with people who have similar problems and are learning to overcome them.

PILES

What are they?

Piles (or haemorrhoids) are veins just inside the back passage, which have become dilated and may cause pain after a bowel movement. They may bleed, and at times become severely inflamed and painful.

What causes piles?

They may be caused by constipation and straining when going to the toilet. Being overweight or pregnant may also be contributing factors. Diarrhoea sometimes aggravates them.

How can piles be prevented?

Avoid becoming constipated by eating a diet high in fibre (fruit, beans, vegetables and cereal products such as bran, wholemeal bread and muesli). See *Nutrition*, section 1.1.

What should you do if they bleed?

Bleeding usually ceases spontaneously when you stop straining. Be very particular about your personal hygiene: bath, or wash the skin around the back passage at least once a day, preferably after opening your bowels. Do not avoid going to the toilet, even if it is painful, as this will make the constipation worse. Piles that protrude should be pushed back inside the back passage by gentle pressure, if possible.

Are piles dangerous?

If bleeding persists over many months you may become anaemic. You should seek medical advice, to ensure the bleeding is from piles and not from some other source. Otherwise they are uncomfortable rather than dangerous.

Will you have to have an operation?

Piles sometimes improve spontaneously if you avoid becoming constipated, or after delivery of the baby, if caused by pregnancy. Sometimes injections are used to 'shrivel up' the piles. Local applications such as witch-hazel or Anusol cream or suppositories may be soothing and help to 'shrink' them. An operation is not usually necessary.

PLEURISY

What is it?

This is the result of inflammation of the lining around the lungs; it often occurs over an area of the lung affected by pneumonia. It causes severe pain in the area on coughing and deep breathing. The treatment is the same as for pneumonia.

PNEUMONIA

What is it?

It is a viral or bacterial infection of a whole lobe or section of a lung, and may be serious enough to need hospital care. It usually follows a cold or other respiratory infection.

What are the symptoms?

- High fever, with rapid shallow breathing.
- Cough, with yellow, green or blood-stained phlegm.
- Pain in the back or side of the chest, often made worse by coughing and deep breathing.

What is the treatment?

If you develop these symptoms you should be under the care of a doctor who will usually prescribe antibiotics such as Ampicillin or Penicillin, and perhaps arrange physiotherapy, if available. While awaiting medical treatment, and through the illness:

- Drink plenty of fluids and stay in bed, or rest comfortably if travelling to where there is medical help.
- Steam inhalations with Friars Balsam, Vick or similar added to the water, will help to loosen the phlegm and open up the lungs again: do this 2 or 3 times daily.
- Take aspirin or paracetamol 4-hourly for the pain and discomfort of the fever.
- Take night-time cough sedatives only: it is best to take an expectorant or nothing during the day, unless coughing is causing a lot of pain. (See section 8.)
- Eat light but regular meals or nourishing drinks. It usually takes a couple of weeks or so to recover from pneumonia and you may

well feel tired for a further couple of weeks. If you have persisting chest pain, this should be checked by a doctor at a follow-up visit.

PSYCHIATRIC PROBLEMS

What are they?
These arise when the proper ordinary functioning of the mind is affected. The problems may be in response to overwhelming stress, and therefore temporary, or they may be recurring or chronic.

Very briefly and basically, psychiatric problems may be divided into neurotic and psychotic groups.

The neurotic group
This includes problems such as anxiety, depression and hysteria (see under separate headings).

The psychotic group
This includes personality disorders and schizophrenia, where there may be a permanent or recurring disassociation from reality. Very skilled help is required to treat or control these conditions.

This book cannot deal with the wide range of possible problems and you should refer to a psychiatrist, a psychologist or to an appropriate book dealing with the subject.

PYELITIS
See *Cystitis*.

RABIES

What is it?
This is an extremely dangerous viral infection (also called hydrophobia), transmitted through the saliva of an infected animal, especially through bites. It is still very common in the Tropics and Sub-Tropics. Bites from rabid stray dogs, cats or, sometimes, jackals, are the commonest source of infection. Thankfully, there is now a very effective vaccination available, although it is still very expensive and not always obtainable. It is being advised for anyone at particular risk: those working with animals, for example.

How can rabies be prevented?
- Control stray dogs and cats.
- Teach children *never* to approach a stray dog or cat.
- If possible, do not keep pet dogs or cats in the Tropics and Sub-Tropics: it is almost impossible to ensure they never have contact with strays. (They also carry many other diseases.) If you must, then **ensure the animal is immunized annually**.
- Any unprovoked attack by a dog or cat, even your own

pet, should be viewed with great suspicion, and immediate medical advice sought. Ensure, if possible, that the animal remains where it can be observed and controlled for the next 10 days.

- Vaccination by the human diploid cell vaccine (also known as the Merieux vaccine):
  2 injections separated by 4 – 6 weeks, followed 6 – 24 months later by a third booster injection.

What is the incubation period?

10 days to 1 year or even longer, but the average is 30 to 50 days. It is shortest in those bitten around the head.

What are the early symptoms?

The virus attacks the nervous system.

In the animal

- Unusual irritability, aggression, restlessness; sometimes only signs of weakness and paralysis.
- Excessive salivation and thirst, but difficulty in swallowing means this cannot be satisfied.

In people

- A short period of depression and general malaise.
- Restlessness, increasing to excitement.
- Fever.
- Excessive salivation.

- Thirst, but again, difficulty with swallowing develops, with painful spasms of the swallowing muscles, eventually making it impossible to drink anything. The spasms are reflexes triggered off by any attempts to drink.

What is the treatment? This must be started as soon as possible after the bite.

- The wounds must be *thoroughly* washed with soap and water, then with any antiseptic solution available (Savlon, Dettol or similar) and with a very strong solution of alcohol (surgical spirit), as 70% alcohol kills the rabies virus it comes into contact with. If the wounds are deep, the washing may need to be done using a fine tube (catheter) inserted into the wounds.
- Ensure the animal is watched carefully, if possible. If it is a stray do not delay the rabies treatment.
- See the table for further advice, but make contact with the local doctors to ensure treatment is available at first signs of rabies in *the animal*.
- Anti-tetanus booster and antibiotics may be necessary for dealing with other infections.

POST-EXPOSURE TREATMENT FOR RABIES
or what to do if you are bitten

10 days after the dog has become infective it will be dead. This means
that if a dog is still alive 10 days after the bite it cannot have been
infected with rabies when it bit you. However, if you are bitten by an
animal *always* go to a hospital for advice even if you have been
vaccinated.

Type of contact with possible rabies	Health of animal at time of contact	Health of animal during next 10 days	Recommended course of action
1. ●No physical contact ●Indirect contact through clothes ●No cuts or abrasions at site of contact	Suspected rabid or definitely rabid	Rabid/dead	No treatment required
2. ●Licks of skin which has cuts or abrasions, however small	(i) Suspected rabid	(a) Remains healthy	Start treatment at once If animal remains healthy, stop treatment
		(b) Becomes rabid	Start treatment at once Complete course of treatment
●Surface scratches or bites	(ii) Rabid animal wild or escaped from observation	Assume rabid if not known	Start treatment at once Complete course of treatment
3. ●Serious deep or multiple bites	Suspected rabid or rabid domestic animal	Assume rabid if not known	Start treatment at once Complete course of treatment unless animal is known to have remained healthy
●Mouth, nose or lips licked by animal	Wild animal or animal escaped from observation		

'RED EYE'
See *Eye problems*.

RHEUMATISM
See *Fibrositis*.

SEXUALLY TRANSMITTED DISEASES

Also known as Venereal diseases or VD
The loneliness and difficulties experienced by many people living in stressful circumstances, or in countries other than their own, may lead to increased sexual temptations. Sexuality is more obvious in some countries, more explicit in talk and imagery, and sexual opportunities may present themselves at moments of low resistance. It is important to be aware of this, but also to have the courage and sense of responsibility to deal with the possible results should you find that you have exposed yourself to the risk of venereal disease.

What is VD?
It is a group of diseases which are transmitted by sexual intercourse. Usually the disease organisms do not survive for long, but gonorrhoea, for example, can be caught from infected towels or toilet seat.

What are the common venereal diseases?

GONORRHOEA
- Very common.
- Caused by the gonococcus bacterium.
- Incubation period in men 2–10 days; in women 7–21 days.
- Causes increased frequency, stinging or burning on passing urine, with a pus-like discharge from the penis or vagina.

In women, if gonorrhoea goes untreated it can lead to infection of the Fallopian tubes (salpingitis) and later infertility.

It is important to note that 60% of infected women have no symptoms but may pass on the disease.

HERPES
- Caused by a herpes virus.
- Incubation period 4–7 days.
- The infection, once established, tends to recur, with relapses occurring at times of other illness or stress.
- Causes small patches of blisters which irritate and sting, and which usually break down to form an ulcer which crusts and heals in about 10 days.

SYPHILIS
- Caused by the organism

Treponema pallidum.

- Has an acute phase with a variety of symptoms, followed by years of symptomless infection eventually leading to severe problems involving the heart and brain which eventually lead to death.
- The first sign is a painless ulcer at the site of entry of the organism into the skin: usually on the penis, the vulva or in the vagina, but may occur in other places.
- The organism does not survive long outside the body, so is unlikely to be caught from toilet seats.

TRICHOMONIASIS

- Usually transmitted sexually, although the organism (Trichonimonas vaginalis) may be carried symptomlessly.
- Men usually have no symptoms and so may carry it and re-infect a partner who has been treated for the illness unless both are treated at the same time.
- In women the infection causes a copious frothy greenish-yellow discharge with soreness of the sexual organs and sometimes also infection higher up in the womb and fallopian tubes.

How should sexually transmitted diseases be treated?

If you suspect that you have caught any form of VD, *do* see a specialist as soon as possible. Some countries have special clinics to deal with it, as the diagnosis and follow-up are important, as is the tracing of all contacts. Despite the embarrassment you may feel in attending a clinic or seeing a doctor, for your own sake as well as that of others, you really must seek help. The treatments are usually oral antibiotics, sometimes injections, and always follow-up. All the types of VD mentioned here are treatable, including herpes. AIDS sufferers can also be helped.
NOTE
Yaws, bejel and pinta are diseases caused by the same type of organism as syphilis, but are not sexually transmitted. They are spread by body contact and are curable with penicillin injections.

AIDS

What is it?

AIDS stands for Acquired Immune Deficiency Syndrome. It is a serious illness caused by a virus that eventually overcomes the body's natural defence system. It may live in the body for 2 years or more before showing any symptoms. It is associated with overwhelming infections, and a particular type of cancer called a Kaposi Sarcoma. It is not necessarily fatal as is sometimes suggested; many do survive.

How is it caught?

It first came to public notice, almost in epidemic proportions, in the homosexual communities of America. It has, however, been in existence for a long time, and is known to exist in Central Africa, for example.

It is spread through body secretions, blood, and blood products. This means that it can be spread through close physical contact, such as sexual intercourse; or through blood transfusions using infected blood; or through blood products such as the treatment given to haemophiliacs. As far as sexual intercourse is concerned, it is the number of sexual partners that appears to be important, so that those with multiple partners, such as prostitutes, some homosexuals, and others with a promiscuous life-style are most at risk.

How can it be avoided?

There is still much research to be done on this illness. There is no specific treatment as yet, nor is there any vaccine against it. Therefore, to avoid contracting the illness, avoid the sort of life-style that puts you at risk.

Correct barrier nursing techniques are essential to ensure as much safety as possible for staff who have to nurse an AIDS victim. It is probably less infectious than hepatitis B, but medical and laboratory staff should take the same precautions.

NOTE

AIDS is not acquired by sitting in the same room, travelling in the same bus, living in the same house, shaking hands with or talking with someone with AIDS.

NON-SPECIFIC URETHRITIS

What is it?

It is a sexually transmitted disease which usually causes itching, discharge and frequency of passing water. It is usually treated with a course of tetracyclines.

SHIGELLOSIS

What is it?

This is an acute infection of the bowel, also known as bacillary dysentery, caused by a group of organisms called shigella. Epidemics may occur in over-crowded conditions with inadequate sanitation. It is particularly common in young children living in such conditions, but it may occur at any age, although it is usually less severe in adults.

How is it spread?

It is spread through cont-aminated food, water and flies.

suffering from it should be nursed in isolation. Any soiled garments need soaking in hot soapy water until they can be boiled.

What are the symptoms?

Sudden onset of diarrhoea, severe abdominal pain (even between bouts of diarrhoea), vomiting and fever. Within the first few days there is blood and mucus mixed with the diarrhoea. It may not be so severe in adults, but diarrhoea may persist for 1–6 weeks.

What is the treatment?

Start fluid replacement at once with small frequent sips of oral rehydration solution (see *Diarrhoea*). Since stool examinations are needed and possibly treatment with antibiotics appropriate for the specific organism, you should call a doctor or travel to a hospital. Continue fluid replacement until you have been seen and advised.

SHINGLES

What is it?

This is caused by a re-activation in an adult of an infection in childhood with the chickenpox virus. This virus attacks the root of a nerve in the spinal column, and causes blisters and an itching or painful rash in a band, usually across one side of the back or

the chest or over a hip, or part of the face. It is only slightly infectious, and tends to attack when you are run down.

Treatment

Acyclovir cream will help, with calamine lotion, pain-killers and patience! It will usually last for 2–3 weeks, but the pain or irritation may last longer.
NOTE
If the rash involves an eye then it is *essential* to get medical help as it can permanently damage the surface of the eye. Some people are left with pain for months or even years after an attack of shingles. Ultrasound treatment sometimes helps; there are also special drugs which may control the pain.

SHORT SIGHT

See *Eye problems*.

SINUSITIS

What is it?

In order to make the bones of the face lighter, there are several pockets or sinuses around the cheek-bones and forehead. These sinuses are lined in the same way that the inside of the nose is, and, when irritated, the lining produces mucus in the same way. This can normally drain away through openings into the nostrils. In an attack of sinusitis there is inflammation of the lining, with infected mucus, which may not drain away.

What are the symptoms?

- Usually a runny nose, or catarrh which has become thick and yellow or green.
- Pain around the nose, eyes, forehead and cheek-bones, with tenderness.
- A heavy congested feeling in the face, especially on bending forwards.
- Often there is a raised temperature and the person feels quite ill.

What is the treatment?

- If the mucus is clear and watery, decongestants such as Actifed ½ – 1 tablet 2 or 3 times a day dry it up and ease the discomfort but beware of drowsiness. (Actifed contains ephedrine and an antihistamine.) Other antihistamines may also help (see section 8) and aspirin or paracetamol will help relieve the pain.
- If the mucus is yellow or green, and there is a lot of tenderness, antibiotics will probably be required to clear the infection. (See section 8.)

SKIN PROBLEMS

ATHLETE'S FOOT

What is it?

This is an infection of the skin caused by a fungus which occurs between the toes, sometimes spreading out to other parts of the foot.

What are the symptoms?

- Itching and burning between the toes.
- Cracks with soreness and redness.
- Scaling, and a spreading rash.

How is it caught?

By walking barefoot over floors or carpets where someone else with athlete's foot has recently walked. The fungus is shed with flakes of skin.

How should it be treated?

- Wash feet thoroughly and dry between the toes using a clean towel each time or paper towels that can be thrown away.
- Apply an antifungal cream such as Clotrimazole (Canesten) or Tolnaftate (Tinaderm) to all affected areas.
- Dust shoes and socks with an antifungal powder, wear clean socks every day, and wash socks and towels very thoroughly.

Repeat this treatment twice daily for at least 3 weeks: all

the infected cells have to be replaced by fresh uninfected cells.

BACTERIAL SKIN INFECTIONS

Small cuts and pricks by sharp objects such as thorns turn septic more readily in warm, moist conditions, such as those experienced in the Tropics, especially if you are also tired and run down, and perhaps, low on Vitamin C.

Cuts, however small, should not be ignored and should be treated with antiseptics such as TCP, salt water soaks, iodine, gentian violet or Savlon, and then kept as clean and dry as possible until healed. Insect bites also become septic more quickly and should be treated in the same way, sooner rather than later, if there is any suggestion of infection developing.

ECZEMA

What is it?

This is often used as a collective name for several types of chronic 'allergic' skin reactions. Dermatitis is a word sometimes used for localized patches or skin reactions to specific substances.

What causes it?

Local patches of inflammation, itching, perhaps flaking and even weeping are usually the result of direct contact with such things as nickel or other metals, elastic or nylon. Some people get a severe dermatitis over the fingers and hands as a result of washing-up liquids and other detergents.

Scattered patches all over the body or in the folds of joints may be caused by certain foods: cow's milk or wheat, for example. Small babies or children tend to suffer from this kind of eczema but adults may also have it. This is generally recurrent unless the cause can be avoided. It may not always be possible to find the cause; sometimes stress makes it worse. It is not the same as psoriasis which is a hereditary condition.

How can one prevent it?

Avoid any known causes. If you have to handle things you know cause an allergic reaction, use barrier creams or rubber gloves.

What is the treatment?

Keep the affected area as clean and dry as possible. Steroid creams or ointments should be used sparingly. Sometimes antihistamines taken regularly will help, as will ultraviolet light (such as sunlight).

Yellow pus weeping or becoming encrusted, with a red inflamed area developing around the patch, indicates a secondary bacterial infection: this may need treatment with antibiotic ointments or medication. Keep it clean and use a mild antiseptic on it twice a day.

IMPETIGO

What is it?
It is a rapidly spreading, very contagious, skin infection, usually caused by the staphylococcus aureus bacterium, which tends to live in the nose. The infection usually starts on the face, but may spread to the rest of the body. It commonly occurs in children.

What does it look like?
Patches of weeping or yellow-crusted sores. The crusted areas are yellow because the fluid leaking from the infected area is pus.

How is it spread?
By nose-picking in the first instance, then by scratching at sores and transmitting the 'bugs' to other areas by touch.

What is the treatment?
● Keep the infected areas clean with TCP or Savlon (which may be mixed with the bath water if the body is involved).
● Use antibiotic ointment on the patches.
● Take a full 7-days course of antibiotics by mouth: Penicillin, Ampicillin, Tetracycline (adults only), Septrin or, if available, Flucloxacillin (for dosages, see *Antibiotics*, section 8).
● Avoid all physical contact with others until 24 hours of antibiotics have been given.

MOLES

What are they?
These are patches of darker pigmentation than the surrounding skin. They may be small or large, flat or raised, pale or dark brown, smooth or hairy. Almost every human being has a few moles.

Do they ever become cancerous?
Very, very occasionally.

What are the symptoms?
Any mole that suddenly changes in any way, by growing bigger or darker, or which bleeds, or becomes inflamed or irritates, should be removed surgically, and examined under the microscope for cancerous changes.

RINGWORM

What is it?
An infection of the skin, scalp or other hairy areas, nails, or any part of the body, which is caused by a fungus.

How is it caught?
By skin to skin contact, or sometimes from infected clothing or animals.

What are the symptoms?
These vary according to the site of the infection. A typical lesion has an irregular, scaling, more-or-less circular edge, with a healing 'fresh-looking' centre. There may be itching and irritation. An infected nail becomes thickened, misshapen, and perhaps crumbly.

What is the treatment?
Apply antifungal creams such as Tinaderm or Canesten after washing. Wear clean clothes each day, keep a towel for your own use only and wash it daily if possible. You will need to do this for about 3 weeks. Some people will also require a specific antifungal drug if the infection is very severe.

SKIN CANCERS

What are the causes?
Most skin cancers arise in skin that has been exposed to the sun either over many years or in short sharp bursts, as in people who go for a couple of weeks to lie in the sun once or twice a year. It is best, when you do go on holiday, to increase the time you spend in the sun gradually over several days: it is the sudden intense exposure that is harmful.

Similarly, intense exposure to ultraviolet light on sunbeds can cause problems.

Skin cancers are very common but they are usually curable.

What to look for
Any new and growing mole, or change in an existing mole, or any spot or ulcer that does not clear up as expected, should be examined by a doctor. It may need to be surgically removed and examined under the microscope to determine the diagnosis.

Treatment
This depends on the site and the type of cancer. Often it is sufficient simply to remove it. Sometimes radiotherapy is also required.

WARTS

What are they?
They are raised irregular or cauliflower-like growths in the skin caused by viruses. They are not cancerous.

Where are they found?
The commonest places are the hands and feet. On the soles of the feet they are called 'verrucas'. Here they appear to grow inwards because the pressure of the body's weight on them pushes them into the sole. They can cause discomfort or pain on walking. They sometimes 'seed'

themselves: smaller warts start growing around the 'parent' one.

How are they caught?
By skin to skin contact with another wart, or skin shed from a wart on to a floor where people may walk barefoot.

How should they be treated?
Warts will often disappear spontaneously. Various 'magic' remedies are supposed to cure them. There are many plasters, paints and lotions which will, with patience, gradually reduce them and perhaps get rid of them without leaving a scar. The common ones contain salicylic acid or formaldehyde which 'kills' the surface layer of cells. The application of the remedy has to be made daily and the top layer removed by gentle use of a pumice stone — it may take many weeks. They can also be frozen, burnt or cut out, but this will leave a scar.

SORE THROAT

What is it?
This is a very common sign of a viral or bacterial infection such as influenza or tonsillitis. It may also be the first sign of a cold.

What is the best treatment?
● Drink plenty of hot soothing drinks, or if you prefer, cold drinks or ice cream.
● Gargle with a solution of 1 teaspoon of salt in a glass of water or with diluted TCP or Savlon.
● Gargle with 2 soluble aspirin every 4 hours if the throat is very sore, and swallow the liquid: you will then get a local soothing effect and the general pain-killing effect of the aspirin.

Taking antibiotics does not cure a sore throat unless it is caused by bacteria, as is often the case in tonsillitis. (See *Tonsillitis*.)

STINGRAY STINGS

The venom of a stingray is in the dorsal spines, which may break off and become partly embedded in the skin. They usually sting as a result of being trodden upon in the sand or shallow water. The pain is intense and immediate, lasting 6–48 hours.

The venom of other poisonous fish is usually carried in special units on the tentacles, and hundreds of units may be fired off into the victim's skin. The pain will depend on the amount of venom received.

What is the treatment?
● Wash thoroughly in the salt

water available.
- Remove any 'bits' that can be seen.
- Treat patient for shock, if necessary (see *First aid*, section 2.3).
- Cover the affected part with the skin of a papaya (pawpaw) — the inside should be against the person's skin. This contains an enzyme which helps to 'dissolve' the 'bits' left in the skin; it also promotes healing and will soothe the pain to some extent.

STROKE

What is it?
It is a sudden paralysis of one or both sides of the body, with or without loss of consciousness.

What causes it?
It may be caused by a blood clot (thrombosis) or a sudden haemorrhage from a blood-vessel in the brain. The result depends on the size of the haemorrhage or the amount of brain tissue that has its blood supply cut off by the clot of blood blocking an artery.

Can it be prevented?
It may not be entirely preventable, but the following helps:
- Maintaining a good healthy diet. (See *Nutrition*, section 1.1.)
- Having your blood pressure checked regularly according to the advice you have been given if you suffer from high blood pressure.
- If you have been given medication to lower your blood pressure, take it regularly: do not stop it without consulting your doctor.

What to do if you think someone has had a stroke
The person should be kept quietly resting until seen by a doctor. To transport him to hospital, see section 3.2.

Can one recover?
Yes, many people do recover completely, or to a great extent. Physiotherapy, patience and optimism, with support from friends and family are all important.

STYE
See *Eye problems*.

SYPHILIS
See *Sexually transmitted diseases*.

TENNIS-ELBOW
See *Joint pains*.

TETANUS

What is it?

It is an illness caused by the tetanus bacterium which lives in soil and in animal faeces. It occurs worldwide. It is sometimes called lockjaw.

How is it caught?

The bacterium may enter through even a small wound; or in newborn babies, through the umbilical cord if it has been cut with a dirty instrument such as a farming implement, or dressed with cowdung as is common in some countries.

What are the symptoms?

The first signs of tetanus do not usually appear until 5–10 days after contact with the bacterium. In some cases they appear as early as 2 days later, or as late as 50 days. They are:

- A stiff jaw with some difficulty in opening is often the first sign; other muscle stiffness may develop.
- Sudden muscle spasms, especially of the back, causing arching as the strong muscles of the back contract: spasms may be triggered off by a sudden movement or noise.
- It becomes increasingly difficult to swallow and breathe, and the spasms cause pain and exhaustion.

What is the treatment?

- The person should be taken to hospital as quickly as possible if lockjaw or muscle stiffness and spasms develop. Hospital care and injections will be necessary.
- On the way to the hospital 1 or 2 people *only* should stay with the patient, to keep him as quiet as possible; if spasms are occurring, protect him from injuring himself on any sharp edges, and speak quietly and soothingly.
- It may not be possible for the person to eat or drink anything.

How can it be prevented?

- Have a course of immunization and maintain regular 5-year boosters.
- Always wash any wounds carefully and thoroughly with antiseptic.
- Use sterile instruments (boiled or passed through a flame) to cut the umbilical cord and use only sterile dressings.
- You can protect your baby by having the tetanus vaccination during pregnancy: this is especially useful if you are likely to have the delivery in an unsterile environment.

TONSILLITIS

What is it?

This is a bacterial infection of one or both tonsils which lie just behind the back of the tongue. The tonsils become swollen and you may be able to see creamy or yellow spots (exudate) on them.

What are the symptoms?

- A sore throat causing difficulty in swallowing.
- Fever.
- Swollen glands, usually those under the jaw.
- Small children often complain of tummy ache and may vomit.

What is the treatment?

- Aspirin or paracetamol (dose according to age) every 4 hours if necessary to control fever and relieve the pain.
- Soothing warm or cold drinks or ice cream.
- Antibiotics (see *Common drugs*, section 8).

NOTE

Ampicillin or Amoxil should not be given in a young adult or teenager in case the illness is glandular fever: if it is, these antibiotics may cause a severe rash. (See *Glandular fever*.)

TOOTHACHE

See *Dental health*.

TRACHOMA

See *Eye problems*.

TRICHOMONIASIS

See *Sexually transmitted diseases*.

ULCERS

See also *Peptic ulcer*.

What are they?

Mouth ulcers are small painful ulcers occurring on the tongue, gums, lips or the palate. They may be caused by viruses, but there are uncertainties as to the exact causes. They tend to occur when a person is run down or has some other infection.

How can they be treated?

- Mouth washes of salt water, TCP or Oraldene may help.
- Take 1,000–2,000mg doses of Vitamin C daily for a couple of weeks.
- Gentian violet 'painted' on to the ulcer 3 or 4 times a day using a cotton wool 'bud', may promote healing, but the colour is a bit off-putting!
- Anaesthetic lozenges, mouthwashes or gels, such as Bonjela, will give temporary relief to enable you to eat.
- Occasionally steroid applications may be used if prescribed by a doctor.

URINARY TRACT INFECTIONS

See *Cystitis*.

VARICOSE VEINS

What are they?

They are veins, usually in the lower part of the leg, which have become 'blown out' and bulging as a result of faulty valves along that section of vein. This may be the result of years of back pressure on the veins due to constipation or obesity; or of pregnancy. The predisposition to varicose veins is sometimes hereditary.

The circulation suffers to some extent, and there may be swelling and aching in the leg as a result.

How can they be prevented?

Avoid constipation and obesity and wear support tights if you are beginning to develop varicose veins.

How are they treated?

- With a high-fibre diet.
- With support tights.
- By injecting the affected veins with something that 'shrivels' them up.
- By 'stripping' the affected veins: this is an operation for which you have to be admitted to hospital.

VENEREAL DISEASES

See *Sexually transmitted diseases*.

VERTIGO

What is it?

It is a sensation of spinning: either the room seems to be spinning around you, or you feel as if you are spinning while the room is stationary. The 'spinning' is often triggered by movements of the head and may be associated with vomiting.

What causes it?

There are many causes. The commonest is a viral infection affecting the balancing organs in the inner ear. There may or may not be an associated upper respiratory infection. This is then known as *labyrinthitis*.

What is the treatment?

This depends on the cause, but Stemetil 5mg 8-hourly or Stugeron 15mg 8-hourly will help to counteract the nausea and some of the giddiness. If it persists or keeps recurring, you should see a doctor.

WARTS

See *Skin problems*.

WORMS

What are they?

There are a large variety of worms that inhabit the human intestine; some cause little or no damage, while others are responsible for a great deal of ill-health. The commonest ones are described here with ways of avoiding them and the treatment, should this be needed.

GROUP 1: THE ROUND WORMS OR NEMATODES

THREADWORMS

(Enterobius vermicularis)
These are extremely common all over the world and occur especially in children. They look like threads of cotton, about ½–1cm long. The adult worms live in the intestine, and may cause quite a bit of itching and irritation around the entrance to the back passage, especially at night. The eggs are passed out in the stools or onto the skin around the anus. They are then swallowed, either by sucking contaminated fingers, biting nails, or with contaminated food. School toilets have sometimes been found to have large numbers of threadworm eggs.

How can they be avoided?

● By ensuring that hands are always carefully washed after using the toilet. Keep toilets clean.

● Avoid drinking water collected from areas likely to be infected.

How can they be treated?

● With Piperazine (mixed with senna) in a mixture called Pripsen. For dosage see *Common drugs*, section 8.

ROUNDWORMS

(Ascaris lumbricoides)
This is a larger worm. The adult may be 15–25cm long, is white or yellow and resembles the common earthworm. Large numbers of roundworms may be present in the intestines, and can cause abdominal pain.

How can they be avoided?

● By ensuring that hands are always carefully washed after using the toilet. Keep toilets clean.

● Avoid drinking water collected from areas likely to be infected.

How can they be treated?

● With Piperazine or Alcopar. For dosage see *Common drugs*, section 8.

HOOKWORMS

(Ankylostoma duodenale and Necator americanus)
These are extremely common in tropical and sub-tropical countries. The adult worms are about 1cm long, and attach themselves to the walls of the

intestine causing chronic blood loss which may lead to anaemia and sometimes chronic diarrhoea.

The eggs are passed out in the stools; if they fall into moist soil they develop into tiny larvae which penetrate the skin. From there they enter the bloodstream, travel through the lungs and eventually reach the intestines and develop into adults.

How can they be avoided?
● Do not walk barefoot near river banks or in any moist areas that may have been used as an 'outside toilet'.

How can they be treated?
Take Bephenium hydroxynaphthoate (Alcopar): see *Common drugs* section 8. Infection with hookworm can only be diagnosed by examination of stools in the laboratory and treatment should be under medical supervision.

GROUP 2: TAPEWORMS
(Cestodes or Flatworms)
There are 3 common varieties: the common beef (taenia solium), the less common pork (taenia saginata) and the fish tapeworm (d. catum). They are acquired by eating imperfectly cooked beef, pork or fish containing the larvae of these tapeworms.

The adult worms are long, flat, white, ribbon-like structures, about 1cm wide and several yards long, subdivided into many segments. Some of these segments break off from time to time and may appear in the stools. The head, the size of a pinhead, is firmly attached to the intestinal wall.

What are the symptoms?
Usually none at all, but sometimes abdominal pains and occasionally abnormal hunger and maybe diarrhoea.

What is the treatment?
This needs treatment in hospital or under medical supervision.

5.2 Men's Section A–Z

CIRCUMCISION

What is it?
This is an operation to remove the foreskin (prepuce) from the tip of the penis. It may be done for religious or medical reasons, usually in childhood but sometimes later.

When is it necessary?
Normally the foreskin separates from the area it protects, the glans, during the first year or two of life. It should not be forcibly pulled back at any time, but the glans should be cleaned when bathing or washing by moving back the foreskin as far as it will go. If, after the first couple of years, it does not pull back fully, circumcision may be necessary, especially if the child develops an infection with a discharge in the space between the foreskin and the glans (balanitis) or has trouble passing urine.

The foreskin exists to protect the glans which is very sensitive, and should not be removed unless there are good reasons for it. It is no longer thought that cervical cancer in women develops less often in societies where circumcision is practised for religious reasons.

IMPOTENCE

What is it?
This is the inability of a man to attain or sustain erection of the penis so that satisfactory sexual intercourse can take place. It is not the same as infertility.

What are the causes?
The causes of impotence are numerous, but are usually psychological. They may be to do with tiredness, anxiety, depression, fear, guilt or resentment towards the partner. Lack of communication between the partners will increase the problem and often leads to deep misunderstandings which only maintain the problem.

Other causes include drugs that lower blood pressure (anti-hypertensive drugs), tranquillizers, and sleeping tablets. Alcoholism, illness of any sort, and chronic illnesses may also cause impotence.

How can it be 'treated'?
- Remember it is usually a temporary problem unless it becomes further compounded by misunderstandings, anxiety or fear.
- Partners: be patient and accepting with each other.
- Talk to each other about

how you feel: if you don't, the scene is set for misunderstandings and hurt.

- If you think it may be the result of a medical problem or of taking medication, talk to a doctor.

Sometimes a psycho-sexual counsellor may be of help, as of course, may any counsellor or friend with whom you can be honest and whom you trust to keep confidences.

Other functional sexual problems, such as premature ejaculation, can often be helped through discussion or psycho-sexual counselling. For your own and your wife's sake, do find someone to talk with about the problem.

INFERTILITY

What is it?
This is not the same as impotence. It is the non-production of sperm by the testicles: the condition may have been present from birth (congenital) or be the result of some illness such as mumps, or of taking certain drugs. It does not usually lead to the inability to function sexually (impotence).

How is it diagnosed?
It can only be diagnosed when the semen is examined under a microscope to count the number of sperm present. In absolute infertility, none are present; in partial infertility, only a small number of normal sperm may be present, perhaps together with some abnormal ones.

Can it be treated?
It is always worth talking the problem over with a specialist, but there is very little that can be done in the case of absolute infertility. However, for the partially infertile there may well be effective treatment.

PROSTATE GLAND ENLARGEMENT

What is it?
The prostate is the gland that sits at the base of the bladder through which the exit tube for urine (the urethra) passes on its way to the penis. The gland produces a liquid which is mixed with semen. Quite a large proportion of men develop enlargement of this gland in their 40s and 50s, and most men will have some degree of enlargement by the time they are in their 60s and 70s.

What are the causes of enlargement?
- By far the commonest is simple benign enlargement which has no specific cause and comes with age.
- The development of a tumour or cancer.

What are the symptoms of enlargement?

● Difficulty in starting to urinate.
● A slow or intermittent stream when urinating and dribbling at the end.
● Having to get up in the night to pass urine several times.

Blood in the urine should be investigated as soon as possible: infection in the urine can cause this, but so can bladder or prostatic tumours.

What is the treatment?

This is usually nothing to start with unless the symptoms are becoming troublesome, or there is any doubt about the possibility of a tumour.

When the symptoms are causing problems, the prostate gland can often be removed through a tube inserted through the penis. This means that recovery is usually quick as there is no abdominal wound to heal.

Impotence or other sexual problems do not usually occur as a result of this operation (prostatectomy).

TESTICLES OR TESTES

What are they?

The testicles or testes are glands enclosed within the scrotum: they produce the sperm which are carried in the duct called the vas deferens from the tube where they are stored, the epididymis, through the prostate into the urethra.

Examination of the testicles

It is important for men to check

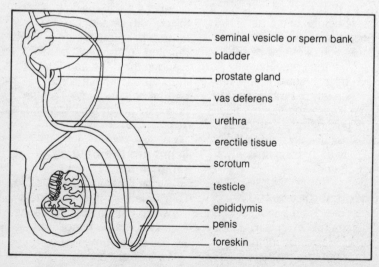

- seminal vesicle or sperm bank
- bladder
- prostate gland
- vas deferens
- urethra
- erectile tissue
- scrotum
- testicle
- epididymis
- penis
- foreskin

their testicles regularly as cysts and tumours may occur here or in the epididymis at any age; if found and dealt with early, even cancers may be treated successfully. Just as women are encouraged to examine their breasts regularly, so men should examine themselves from time to time, and ask for a medical examination if they find any changes, such as swelling or tenderness.

Some causes of swellings in the scrotum

A cyst is a collection of fluid which commonly occurs in the epididymis, above the testicle. It is usually benign and may remain unchanged for years, or may require an operation.

A varicocele is a cystic swelling of the blood vessels which form a network around the vas deferens. It is also benign and may be unchanged for years, causing no problems.

A hernia is a pouch protruding into the scrotum from a weakness in the groin region; its contents are a part of the bowel which pushes through the weakness because of increased pressure in the abdomen.

It may be caused by the sort of straining that occurs in heavy lifting, or it may be a weakness that has been present from birth. In the latter case the hernia will be present although not necessarily noticed, from birth, and will probably be dealt with by operation during childhood.

A tumour is a solid growth which usually develops in the testicle. It may be benign or malignant, but must always be dealt with as soon as possible in case it is malignant.

NOTE

Those who have had undescended or partially descended testicles should ensure that they examine themselves every 6 months or so, as the risk of developing cancer is higher in these cases.

A tender swelling in the skin of the scrotum may be an infection in one of the oil-producing glands (sebaceous) at the base of a hair follicle. This can be treated with a solution of salt or with TCP bathing and Savlon cream; sometimes antibiotics may be necessary and the sebaceous cyst may need to be removed.

Orchitis is an infection which causes swelling and tenderness in one or both testicles, and is usually accompanied by general malaise and fever. It may be viral, such as in mumps, or bacterial, and is usually treated with antibiotics. It is best to get medical advice if possible. If medical advice is not immediately available, treat as follows:

● Rest in bed.

- Bathe the scrotum several times daily in tepid water to cool and soothe.
- Support the scrotum with a loose bandage so as to hold it gently.
- Take 2 aspirin or 2 paracetamol 4-hourly.
- Take Ampicillin 250mg 6-hourly for 7 days or Septrin 2 tablets twice daily for 7 days.

In a child under 12, adjust the dosage of aspirin or paracetamol and antibiotics according to age. (See also *Antibiotics* and *Common drugs*, section 8.)

Orchitis may result in infertility, but this is by no means inevitable.

VASECTOMY

What is it?
This is an operation to block the passage of sperm down the duct in each testicle (the vas deferens). It is usually done under local anaesthetic. It involves making 2 small cuts on either side of the scrotum, finding, cutting and tying off the cut ends of the vas deferens on each side. It does not usually lead to impotence or other sexual problems. The semen has to be examined 3 months after the operation to check that the operation has been successful. Until then other methods of contraception have to be used to prevent pregnancy.

Are the results permanent?
Usually, although some surgeons will try to reverse the operation in special circumstances. The success rate of reversal operations is not very good.

5.3 Women's Section: A–Z

BREAST CANCER

What is it?
Breast cancer is any type of malignant growth or tumour in one or both breasts.

Can it be cured?
If found and treated early enough, it can be cured. It is therefore very important for every woman to know how to examine her breasts, and to ask for a medical examination as quickly as possible if she finds a lump or any persistent change in either breast. Women who take the contraceptive pill should ask a doctor to examine them once a

year and it is a good idea for all women to have a regular check-up.

Breast examination

The basic rules are:

- Get to know yourself; know what your breasts normally feel like at different times of the menstrual cycle.
- If you notice any change that persists more than a couple of weeks, and, in particular, does not disappear after your period, arrange to see a doctor as soon as possible.
- If you notice any lump that feels separate from the mass of breast tissue, ask a doctor to examine you, within days if possible: lumps, painful or not, are not usually cancerous, but they should always be examined.
- If your nipple produces a discharge of any sort, and, in particular, if there is any blood, you must be examined within a couple of days.
- If one breast becomes bigger than the other, or one nipple starts turning inwards instead of protruding normally, see a doctor.

What should my breast feel like?

A normal breast consists of fatty tissue mixed with breast tissue hanging together in an irregular mass. It goes through certain changes every month, and some women are more conscious of these changes than others. Sometimes the changes become more marked for a few months and then settle down again. The changes are due to changing levels of hormones in the bloodstream and are as follows:

- Just after a period: the breast usually feels soft and unlumpy, with no tenderness or swelling.
- At mid cycle, around ovulation, there may be some swelling of the breast tissue, perhaps some lumpiness and tenderness, especially up towards the arm.
- During the week or so before the period there may be increased swelling, lumpiness and tenderness, with the nipple rather sensitive and perhaps more erect than usual.

Become familiar with your own cycle of changes, and what your breasts feel like at these times.

How to examine your breast

There are many methods: the following is a simple one to remember, but first note:

- Always use the right hand for the left breast and the

left hand for the right breast.

- Always use the flat of your hand and fingers, not the tips of your fingers.
- Ensure you are warm and comfortable, and unlikely to be disturbed, and that you can lie down flat.
- Have a mirror available at chest level.
- Examine your breasts after a period when they are least likely to be lumpy.
- Some people advise monthly examinations; the important thing is that you remember to do it at least every 3 months; if you are likely to forget, then do it monthly.

The actual examination

- Lie down comfortably on a bed or sofa with both arms by your side and relaxed.
- Think of your breast as a circle with the nipple as the centre.
- Use your right hand to examine your left breast, starting at the centre and, with the flat of your fingers, working your way outwards in a circular fashion keeping them relaxed to follow the curve of the breast.
- Move the whole breast over your ribs as you feel your way round, and make sure you have felt right up towards the collar bone: here the ribs feel solid and can be followed outwards from the central chest bone (sternum).
- Feel up into the armpit on the side you are examining: push up into it as far as you can, then come down the side of the breast using the flat of your fingers and the same circular movements, moving the tissue over the ribs (the part of the breast going up into the armpit is called 'the tail').
- With the tips of your fingers this time, feel just around the nipple with gentle movements so that you feel the ducts which come up from the deeper breast tissue and surface at the nipple: any blockage in a duct will be felt as a tiny lump.
- Finally, stand in front of the mirror and look at your breasts: are they smooth, more or less the same size, and do they look the same as they have always done?

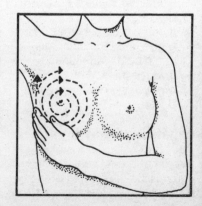

What does a breast lump feel like?

There are different sorts of lump: some are solid and feel like a nut, some are 'cystic' and feel like a pea; usually they move under your fingers and feel somehow separate and different from the other breast tissue.

Are breast lumps always cancerous?

No! Most lumps do not turn out to be cancerous: these are called 'benign'. They can be easily removed, if necessary, for examination under a microscope to make absolutely sure. Even cancerous lumps, if found early enough, may be removed only from where they occur, leaving the rest of the breast intact. Sometimes it is necessary to remove the whole breast (mastectomy). If the lump is cancerous, you will also be given radiotherapy treatment and regular follow-ups for many years. Many women who have been treated for cancer of the breast have survived happily for as long as anyone else might have done.

MENSTRUAL PROBLEMS

What is menstruation?

It is the bleeding which occurs regularly from puberty until the menopause. Each individual has her own pattern but it usually occurs every 4-6 weeks. It happens as a result of the build-up of the lining of the womb as it prepares to receive a fertilized egg. If the egg implants in the lining, it will develop into a baby. If no egg implants, the lining is shed and bleeding occurs. The whole process is controlled by a complicated and sensitive hormone system.

The first day of bleeding in one 'period' to the first day of the next 'period' is called one cycle.

How much bleeding is 'normal'?

Every woman is different, but most women bleed for between 3-6 days, with heavier bleeding on the first day or two, sometimes accompanied by cramping pains felt low down in the abdomen.

A 'normal' loss means changing sanitary towels or tampons every 2-4 hours; some lose more and find their 'protection' soaked within an hour: this would be called heavy bleeding, especially if she also loses clots of blood. Some bleed very lightly for only a day or two. (Those who take the contraceptive Pill find that their 'periods' are usually much lighter than before starting to take it.) If there is a dramatic change in your particular pattern, you should seek medical advice.

Painful periods

This condition, also known as dysmenorrhoea, refers to the spasmodic lower abdominal pain with backache which sometimes occurs before or soon after bleeding starts. It may last for a few hours or a couple of days. It is sometimes accompanied by nausea and a feeling of faintness.

It is caused by a build up of hormones known as prostaglandins in the lining of the womb and it is made worse by constipation.

Treatment is as follows:

- Aspirin or paracetamol 2 tablets 4-hourly, with either a hot-water bottle and rest or exercise!
- In severe cases, stronger tablets, such as Mefanamic acid (Ponstan 250mg — see *Common drugs*, section 8) may be necessary. It is a good idea to start 1 – 2 days *before* the onset of the period as this will reduce the prostaglandin levels. Take 1 capsule 3 times per day for 1 – 2 days, then 2 capsules 3 times per day as soon as bleeding starts, for 2 – 3 days.
- If the above does not work you may need a different anti-prostaglandin (see *Common drugs* section 8), or one of the hormone treatments.

Irregular periods

Irregular, scanty or absent periods (not due to pregnancy) are a common occurrence when any major change occurs, such as travelling or moving to a new country. Don't worry — after a few months your usual pattern will become re-established again. If things are not back to normal after 6 months, do discuss it with your doctor.

Pre-menstrual tension

Women who suffer from pre-menstrual tension (or the pre-menstrual syndrome as it is also called) notice that for a few days, or anything up to 2 weeks before their period is due, they become increasingly tired, tense, irritable, and perhaps weepy and depressed. Some women also find they are much more clumsy in their movements and are more likely to have accidents during this time. Some have physical symptoms, such as headaches, swollen ankles and back-ache, and some gain several pounds in weight, which they lose as soon as the period has started. This gain in weight is due to fluid retention, which may also contribute to the feeling of depression. Some women find they change completely in character in the week or two before a period, so that their families can always tell when one is due, and keep out of their way! Much research is being done into the causes of this problem and as yet it is not fully understood. However, the hormone changes that are taking place during the menstrual cycle undoubtedly do cause some of the problems; there seems to be a deficiency of the hormone progesterone in some women, and in some a deficiency of vitamin B6.

The following may help ease pre-menstrual tension:

- Reduce your coffee and tea intake to a maximum of 3 cups of either per day.
- Reduce your salt intake: for at least the 2 weeks leading up to the period, add *no* salt to your food.
- Increase your vitamin B6 intake (see *Nutrition*, section 1.1 for natural sources): yeast tablets also give a low dose, and vitamin B6 tablets are available in dosages from 5mg to 100mg. Some women need 100–150mg daily, but do not exceed this dose as it may be toxic in overdosage.

If none of this helps, consult a doctor: you may need drugs to help you pass water more often (diuretics) which will reduce your fluid retention, or hormone treatment.

Heavy periods

Some women lose large volumes of blood during menstruation, and 'flooding' sometimes occurs, when the blood pours out, rather like having a tap turned on. Some women also lose clots of blood. If you are losing enough blood to soak through a sanitary towel every hour or less you should see a doctor for examination and advice. You may become anaemic and need iron tablets, as well as treatment to stop the heavy bleeding.

There are a variety of causes for heavy periods, including hormone imbalance and benign lumps of tissue that develop from the muscle in the womb (fibroids). Paracetamol 2 tablets 6–8 hourly may reduce the flow to some extent. There are also stronger drugs which a doctor can prescribe, and fibroids can be removed by operation.

THE MENOPAUSE

What is it?

It means, literally, the ending of menstruation. It commonly occurs between the ages of 48 and 53, but may occur earlier or later. Women often seem to have the same pattern as their mothers.

What causes it?

The ovaries, which up till now have been producing the eggs (ova) every month, and with them, certain hormones, especially the oestrogens, are gradually 'shutting down' the production. The 'shut down' usually occurs over a period of years so that there are no sudden dramatic changes except for the cessation of periods.

What are the symptoms?

For some lucky women all that happens is that the periods just stop. However, most women experience a variety of symptoms which include some of the following, the most common being at the top of the list:

- Scanty or irregular bleeding (heavy flooding is not usually due to the menopause, and should be investigated).
- Hot flushes — the commonest symptoms — (when the face and neck suddenly become flushed and red, often followed by profuse sweating lasting for a few minutes).
- Tiredness.
- Dizziness.
- Headaches.
- Insomnia, often due to profuse night-sweats.
- Anxiety and depression (which may have other causes too).
- Irritability.
- Joint and muscle pains.
- Palpitations.
- 'Pins and needles' in hands and feet.

Another common problem is a feeling of dryness in the vagina which may cause soreness and make sexual intercourse difficult. This may be helped by using KY jelly for lubrication, or hormone creams (after discussion with a doctor) which will improve the condition of the lining of the vagina.

After the menopause, women's bones become lighter and more brittle. This is caused by the low oestrogen levels, but other associated factors may be a poor diet, poor absorption of calcium, a vitamin D deficiency and lack of exercise.

How can these problems be minimized?

- Maintain an active and out-going lifestyle.
- Maintain a good balanced diet (see sections on nutrition and health maintenance).
- Do some regular exercise.

If the symptoms are interfering with your life, and particularly if you are becoming depressed or having some difficulties (with sexual intercourse, for example) do discuss the problems with a doctor. There are hormone creams that can be prescribed for the vaginal dryness, tablets that will control, if not eliminate, the hot flushes, and there is hormone replacement therapy, if necessary.

What is hormone replacement therapy?

This means artificially replacing the hormones which are no longer being produced normally by your body. This can be done by injection, implants or more commonly, by daily tablets of a combination of hormones arranged in the same sort of pattern that the ovaries would have produced. It is like taking the contraceptive Pill, and there will even be a return of some regular bleeding, just as before the menopause.

If you are on hormone replacement therapy (HRT) you should have the following check-ups:

- Monthly breast-checks (done by yourself).
- Annual breast examination by a doctor.
- Six-monthly blood-pressure checks.
- Annual internal examinations and cervical smears.

The same applies to women using oestrogen creams regularly as the oestrogen is absorbed into the bloodstream.

MISCARRIAGE

See section 7.

PREGNANCY

See section 7.

SALPINGITIS

What is it?

It is an infection of the Fallopian tubes (the salpinges), the tubes through which the eggs pass from the ovaries to the womb. The inflammation caused by the infection may cause blockage of the tubes, leading to later problems with fertility.

What causes it?

There are many organisms that can cause this, including gonorrhoea and trichomonas vaginalis (see *Sexually transmitted diseases*). Many are not sexually transmitted, but live in the area, or have reached it through the bloodstream.

What are the symptoms?

- Pain in the lower abdomen, on one or both sides.
- Sometimes a vaginal discharge.
- Fever, low-grade, or coming on from time to time, preceded by shivering.
- Back-ache.
- General feeling of ill-health, perhaps nausea and loss of appetite.

What is the treatment?

- You should see a doctor for an internal examination and diagnosis if you suspect you have this.
- It needs treatment with antibiotics as soon as

possible to reduce the risk of blocked tubes.

- You will need to rest and perhaps take pain-killers during the treatment.

THRUSH

What is it?
It is an infection caused by a yeast which lives in the digestive system and in the vagina. It can become an infection when a person is run down and tired, has influenza or other illnesses, or is taking antibiotics. The common sites of infection are the mouth and the vagina.

What are the symptoms and signs?
In the mouth, a thick white deposit can be found on the tongue or cheeks, with soreness. This is common in babies but can occur at any age.

In the vagina, thrush causes the formation of a thick white or creamy discharge (sometimes likened to yoghurt or cream cheese) with itching and soreness.

How is it treated?
In the mouth, it is usually treated with Nystatin Oral Suspension: ½ – 1ml after meals or drinks.

In the vagina: pessaries (Nystatin, Canesten for example) and a soothing cream are used to treat the condition. Sometimes the old-fashioned remedy of gentian violet will cure it if started early, but it causes staining of underwear. Soak the tip of a tampon and insert 2 or 3 times a day. Do not douche.

How can it be prevented?
Thrush has a tendency to recur at times of stress, but if treated at the first signs of infection (itching, usually) it can often be controlled quickly. Avoid wearing tight clothes (such as jeans) and nylon tights: cotton, being more absorbent, is much better. Bathe or wash daily, or more often if very hot and sweaty, but do *not* add Dettol (or other antiseptic) to the water and **do not douche**: this tends to make it worse and causes other problems. Bubble baths also tend to increase the problem.

Partners should be treated simultaneously to prevent re-infection. The cream may be applied to the penis.

5.4 Children's Section: A–Z

ASTHMA IN CHILDHOOD
(See also *Wheezing*.)

What is it?
Children with asthma have repeated attacks of wheezing or coughing, and find it difficult to breathe out. Sometimes the chest feels very tight but not much wheezing is heard: this is because it is difficult for the air to move in and out of the tubes at all. The chest is quite normal between attacks. It is not usually called asthma until a child has had 2 or more attacks.

What causes the wheezing?
- Spasm of the muscles and narrowing of the air-tubes.
- Swelling of the lining of the tubes.
- Sticky mucus 'plugging' the tubes.

What triggers an attack?
- Allergies to such things as house dust and the house dust mite, or animal fur.
- Breathing in a large amount of these: during the night, for example, in the bed-clothes.
- Infections, usually caused by viruses.
- Emotion, excitement, fear.
- Exercise, especially in cold weather.
- Irritants, especially tobacco or cigarette smoke, or air pollution.

Can asthma be cured?
No. The person who has asthma has particularly sensitive lungs, so there will always be the tendency or possibility that an attack may occur if the right trigger-factors are present. However, it is possible to control it, and often it is possible to prevent attacks.

Do children grow out of it?
Some do: more than half of the children suffering with asthma will grow out of it before the age of about 10. About a third will grow out of it but may find it returns in later life, while about one fifth continue to have asthma all their lives.

Do such factors as diet and climate affect asthma?
Yes, both may do. Children who are totally breast-fed for at least the first 3 months of life are less likely to develop asthma, and there is a small number of children who are allergic to foods such as cow's milk, eggs and some meats. You would need expert advice about the diagnosis and diet; changes in the weather may

affect a child with asthma: for example, wind changes may bring more pollen into the area, and cause a reaction.

Is exercise dangerous?
No, but the child is usually a good judge of how much or how little he can do. Emotional excitement associated with the exercise will also increase the likelihood of an attack of asthma being induced. Do not encourage a child to be an invalid. Use the treatment prescribed wisely to counteract the tendency of exercise to induce an attack. Some medication such as Intal (sodium cromoglycate) will reduce the tendency if used *regularly*, and increase the ability to do more exercise: some Olympic runners use this!

What is the treatment of asthma in childhood?
The child will be best helped by the parents and the doctor working together. Treating each separate attack of asthma only deals with the immediate situation, but does nothing for the future of the child.

Aim first of all at preventing attacks, then treating them if they occur in spite of this.

How to prevent an asthma attack
Avoid the trigger-factors, or take the treatment *before* the trigger-factor triggers an attack! For example, take the relevant medicine before the child is about to do a race.

Use one of several possible medications: each child will be different. The medications include, for example, salbutamol syrup (Ventolin) 5ml 3 times per day, or salbutamol inhaler, which opens the tubes in a spasm, or sodium cromoglycate inhaler (Intal) which stops the tendency to spasm if used regularly 2–4 times daily.

Tablets and syrups may be vomited up. If vomited within 10 minutes of giving them, wait for a short while and give a second dose.

Inhalers must be used properly: the mist or spray must be carried *into* the air-tubes on the breath to be effective. Children can learn to do this as early as 3–4 years old.

Treatment of an attack
Salbutamol or Aminophylline are often used to treat an asthma attack. These are given through a nebulizer: a simple device which creates a mist out of the fluid medicine. The mist can be breathed in through a mask. The nebulizer works on a footpump or electricity, and is very useful to have at home if you have an asthmatic child.

A spacer or nebuhaler also releases a spray of medicine

into a wide chamber. The patient can breathe in the mist from the chamber rather than having to breathe in at the same time as pressing the inhaler 'pump', which some find difficult.

Either of these methods may be used to treat an acute attack, but if the spasm is not relieved, it may be necessary to insert an Aminophylline suppository, or a doctor may give an injection into a vein. Sometimes the child has to go to hospital.

The use of steroids
Steroids are very powerful drugs, and should only be used under strict medical supervision. Do not stop taking them suddenly; the dosage should always be tailed off gradually. Any doctor treating someone taking steroids should be told that they are being taken, or have been taken recently.

Should the child have antibiotics during each attack?
No, not necessarily. Many attacks are triggered by viruses, against which there are as yet no effective antibiotics. When an attack is triggered by exercise or emotion, there is clearly no need for them.

Is there anything else that helps?
Some people find acupuncture, homoeopathy or hypnosis effective. Humidifiers, iodizers and dust extractors have not proved helpful.

BED-WETTING
The age at which a child becomes fully 'potty-trained' and therefore 'dry' varies a great deal, and most children will continue to have the occasional wet night till the age of 4 or 5.

An older child who is bed-wetting frequently should have a check-up by a doctor. It doesn't help, and may make matters much worse, to become angry or to punish the child. He or she simply does not wake up at all or until it is too late.

What are the causes?
Bed-wetting may be caused by upheaval and changes, or some emotional disturbance, or, if recurring more frequently, with an infection of the urine which needs treatment.

There may also be some other medical or neurological problem.

Simple measures to try
Do not give the child anything to drink for 2 hours before bedtime and ensure he or she uses the toilet just before going to bed. Wake the child up to

go again just before you yourself go to sleep. Put the child on the potty in the night, if you are awake, or set an alarm to wake him to pass urine every 2 hours. It may also be possible to change the child's body rhythm (biological or diurnal rhythm) to pass more urine in the mornings by giving him more fluids to drink in the mornings, and restricting them in the evenings.

If these measures fail

Ask a doctor to examine the child. He may do some investigations, offer some medication or suggest an 'enuresis alarm', a buzzer which is activated by the first drop of urine passed, waking the child — hopefully! — and you.

BEHAVIOUR PROBLEMS

What are the causes?

These are usually to do with some emotional disturbance associated with change and upheaval. They may indicate a deep sense of insecurity, or jealousy, perhaps of a new baby. They may be the result of tensions between the parents, or anxieties and fears the parents are feeling: children pick up 'vibrations' very quickly, even if nothing has been said.

Very strict discipline with no explanations to the child may also result in eventual rebellion and behaviour problems such as refusal to eat or sleep. A child who understands the reasons for certain rules will find it much easier to follow them, at least for some of the time! Try to avoid making mealtimes into a battle-field; make bedtime a good time with stories and good-night kisses and cuddles.

Sometimes a general low level of health may result in an irritable, badly-behaved child, and a check-up may be advisable. There is also some evidence that certain foods or chemicals can cause behaviour problems: additives in processed food may be to blame. If you suspect a certain food, cut it out *completely* for 2 weeks, then re-introduce it and watch what happens. If the child improves when the food is taken out of the diet but gets worse again when it is re-introduced, then this could be the answer, and it would be sensible to avoid that food or particular additive. See *Food allergies*.

Bringing up children, even in ideal situations, is never easy; parents can learn from each other. Sometimes specialist help may be needed, and it may not just be the child who needs the help! Family therapy is often of great value in this situation.

BREATH-HOLDING ATTACKS

What are they?

These usually occur between the ages of 1 and 4. They are triggered by a sudden shock or fright, or by a temper tantrum, where a lot of yelling and screaming has occurred. The child holds his breath for about 20 seconds, becomes blue and then suddenly falls over, apparently unconscious, and starts breathing again. If there is any loss of consciousness, it is quickly regained, and there are no jerking movements as in a 'fit' or convulsion.

What is the treatment?

None. Do not allow your fear of such attacks to force you into giving in to the temper tantrums. When the tantrum is over, talk to the child about what has happened, and about why he was in such a temper. Being able to talk about the frustration that brought it on, and having clear firm explanations given as to why you did not allow him to have what he wanted, will eventually help to reduce the frustration levels. But a great deal of patience is needed.

If you are concerned that the child is not well or back to normal after an attack, see a doctor.

BREATHING PROBLEMS

See also *Asthma, Croup, Wheezing*.

MOUTH BREATHING

What are the causes?

If a child is breathing only through the mouth, this is often the result of a blocked nose either through a cold, allergic rhinitis and hay fever, or through enlarged adenoids.

Mouth breathers tend, perhaps, to be more prone to throat and nose infections.

What can be done?

Adenoids are glands (of the tonsil variety) which are situated at the back of the junction of the nose and pharynx, and if they are blocking normal breathing through the nose it may be advisable to have them removed. This needs to be discussed with an ear, nose and throat (ENT) specialist, but tonsils and adenoids are only removed if there are very strong signs of chronic infection; even then they are usually left if possible to the age of 7 or older.

CHICKEN POX

See *Common childhood illnesses*.

COLIC IN BABIES

What is it?

Some small babies develop severe gripping or spasmodic tummy pains especially towards the evening. This causes them to cry a lot and to pull up their legs or curl up in pain. There is no vomiting, usually, and the baby is otherwise quite well. It is important to have the baby checked by a doctor, however, to ensure there is no illness and that the weight is going up steadily.

What is the treatment?

Gripe water or 1 teaspoonful of Merbentyl 15 minutes before feeds may help. Always ensure the baby has been properly 'burped', and if he is constipated, add (if bottle-fed) a teaspoonful of brown sugar to the feeds, and give extra water between them in any case.

Carry the baby close to you in a sling: this will comfort the baby, but leave your hands free to get on with other things.

If you bottle-feed the baby, it is possible that the milk doesn't agree with him. A change from a cow's milk formula to goat's milk or soya milk may be necessary. If you do try goat's milk, ensure that it has been properly boiled before giving it to the baby. It may not have been sterilized or pasteurized, even if cow's milk usually is

where you live.

Sometimes, in breast-fed babies, the mother's diet affects the baby. Coffee, alcohol, or certain foods or medicines may be to blame.

Patience and the knowledge that the colic will settle eventually, will help. It doesn't usually continue to recur after about 3 months.

CONSTANT COUGHS AND COLDS, OR RUNNY NOSE

What are the causes?

These are sometimes due to an allergic reaction, such as hay fever, and not an infection at all. Sometimes it is pollen and house dust that is responsible and antihistamines such as Phenergan or Piriton will help control the conditions, though not cure it.

Some nose sprays, such as Ephedrine and Otrovine Paediatric are good. They should not be used for more than one week, as they do cause 'rebound' swelling after a while. This means that the lining of the nose swells as soon as the drops are stopped, and the runny nose starts again.

Some foods, such as cow's milk or wheat may also be responsible in some children:

see *Food allergies*.

If your child has a constantly runny nose or a constant cough, you should take him to be examined by a doctor.

CONSTIPATION IN BABIES

What is it?
Difficulty in passing a stool or stools that are small and solid.

What is the treatment?
More fluids are needed. Give the baby 2 or 3 ounces of extra boiled water (flavoured if you like) between each feed. You can also add a teaspoon of brown sugar to the water or to his feed (if bottle feeding): this will help to soften the stool.

CROUP

What is it?
This is the barking, harsh cough that children get when they have an inflammation of the voice-box or vocal cords (laryngitis). Some children are much more prone to it than others and an attack may come on very suddenly. It is frightening for both the parents and the child, as there is usually also some feeling of difficulty in breathing, and a hoarse voice.

What you can do
Don't panic: your panic will frighten the child and perhaps worsen the breathing difficulty. Instead:

- Steam up the room as quickly as possible by, for example, running the hot water in the bathroom with the doors shut, or boiling several pans of water, and take the child into the steamy atmosphere. This will relieve some of the swelling and make the cough and breathing easier.
- If there is real difficulty in breathing in spite of the steam treatment, call a doctor or go to the nearest hospital at once; try to keep calm and be re-assuring towards the child.
- If breathing is not a problem, a dose of aspirin or paracetamol (see *Common drugs*, section 8, for correct dosage), with the steam treatment, will help. Breathing in the steam from a bowl of hot water will be more effective, if the child is old enough to do this. If the child's temperature is also high, remove the clothes and sponge all over with tepid water to reduce the temperature.
- If the temperature and cough continue into the next day, a doctor should examine the child; antibiotics may be needed to deal with the infection. An attack often occurs at night and the child may be much

better by the next morning. It frequently recurs for several nights with trouble-free days between.

DIARRHOEA

See also general section on *Diarrhoea* (see page 104). The important thing to do for anyone with diarrhoea, and *especially* babies and young children, is to **replace the fluid loss** by giving small *frequent* sips of water or oral rehydration fluid. If the child is vomiting or refusing to take fluids, it has to be fed spoonful by spoonful more or less continuously. Rice water may also be used and may help to thicken the stool and to stop the diarrhoea a bit sooner.

Signs of 'drying out' in a child

- In babies, a sunken fontanelle (the 'soft spot' in the skull).
- Dry tongue.
- Dark circles around the eyes, especially underneath.
- Very dark yellow (that is, concentrated) urine; small quantities or none at all.
- Excessive drowsiness.
- Skin that does not spring back flat when pinched up.

Any combination of these means that more fluid is being lost than replaced; increase the frequency of the sips of fluid and continue giving fluids while taking the child to the nearest hospital or doctor. Diarrhoea and vomiting in children are often signs of infections elsewhere, such as ears and throat. These are often of viral origin, so do not necessarily require antibiotics.

DIPHTHERIA

See *Immunizations in children* and *Common childhood illnesses*.

EARACHE WITH FEVER

See also *Ear problems*, section 5.1.

What are the causes?

Earache is caused by inflammation of the ear-drum, with or without collection of fluid behind it. The fluid collects because the Eustachian tube, connecting the back of the ear to the back of the nose, becomes blocked due to swelling of the tissues around it. It is very common in children, and is usually associated with a cold, sore throat or cough. Some children are more prone to earache than others.

What are the symptoms?

- Pain in the affected ear. A child who is not yet able to speak will pull at the ear, and perhaps also bang it or push it into a pillow. The earlobe may be reddened as a result.

- Signs of a cold: runny or blocked nose.
- Usually, a rise in temperature.
- Vomiting and diarrhoea sometimes accompany ear infections.

What is the treatment?

If there is a raised temperature, with a runny nose, sore throat, hoarse voice, and especially if the child is vomiting and has enlarged glands in the neck:

- Ask a doctor to examine the child if possible; antibiotics may be needed.
- Give aspirin or paracetamol every 4 or 6 hours to reduce the pain and the temperature.
- Actifed syrup (or another decongestant) and Ephedrine nosedrops 3 times a day will help to open up the Eustachian tube and allow the fluid to drain away. It will also dry up the runny nose.
- If you do not have access to a doctor, but are sure the signs are clear that the child has an ear infection, give him a full 5–7 day course of Ampicillin or Septrin (see *Common drugs*, section 8).

EARACHE WITHOUT FEVER

If there is no fever and the child is otherwise well:

- Give a dose of aspirin or paracetamol.
- There may be hard wax in the ear causing pain with deafness: olive oil drops 3 times a day for 3 or 4 days will soften this and help clear it. **Do not use cotton buds to 'clean' inside the ear**. You may perforate the ear-drum or pack the wax in harder.
- Another cause of earache is inflammation of the outer canal which leads to the ear-drum. This may be caused by an eczema-like condition, or by the sensitive lining reacting to such things as chlorine in swimming pools. See a doctor if the pain is severe or recurring.
- Ask a doctor to examine the child, if the pain persists. A small child may have put something like beads or stones into his or her ears: **Do not attempt to remove these yourself**.
  See further under *Hearing problems, Perforated ear-drums,* also *First aid*.

If there are frequent, recurring earaches, with a more or less continuously runny nose, and perhaps deafness:

- Ask a doctor to examine the child: he or she may be developing 'glue ears', and need special medication to soften the sticky, gluey fluid that has formed; sometimes a small operation to provide drainage is necessary.

● The child may be allergic to something inhaled in the air or eaten regularly. Some children are allergic to cow's milk or some cereals, for example, and it may be worth trying to experiment with avoiding suspected foods completely for 2 weeks, then re-introducing them and seeing whether the child improves and then becomes worse again.

EXCESSIVE CRYING IN BABIES

What are the causes?
Babies, having not yet acquired the skill of language, have only limited ways of expressing their feelings! Crying may express discomfort, hunger, pain, misery, anger, loneliness: in fact, anything he is not happy about! Discomfort may be caused by wet nappies, or by being too hot or too cold. He may just be saying, 'I'm here; please notice me!'

Excessive crying usually indicates some acute pain, such as colic, earache, or teething pain, and dealing with the cause may be what's needed. A paracetamol mixture such as Calpol is useful to keep in stock, and a dose might help to settle the

problem. If it doesn't, ask a doctor to check the baby.

EYE PROBLEMS

CONJUNCTIVITIS
This is very common, especially with colds or if the child is unwell in some other way (with measles, for example). The white of the eye becomes red and inflamed, and there is a sticky yellow discharge from the eye when the infection is caused by bacteria.

If there is only watering of the eye, the cause may be an allergy (when usually both eyes are involved), a speck of dust or splinter or similar in the eye, or a viral infection. It is best to ask a doctor to examine and advise about treatment.

In the absence of a doctor
● Mix ¼ teaspoon (5ml) of salt with ½ cup (100ml) of cooled boiled water.
● Clean the eyelids with sterile cotton wool soaked in this solution. Use one piece of cotton wool for one eye, wiping from the inner corner to the outer. Discard that piece and take a fresh one for the other eye.
● In older children, the eye can be bathed by 'blinking' it into an egg cup full of the solution. This will soothe the

irritation and is a mild antiseptic and can be used as frequently as necessary. If it has not cleared the infection in 2 or 3 days, or if it is obviously becoming worse, you will need antibiotic drops or ointment.

SQUINTS

It is very common for a baby to look as though it has a mild squint, due to a broad nose and an eye-fold over the inner corner of the eye. If the two pupils do not move together in parallel, ask a doctor to check. The sooner the treatment for a squint can be started the better, and advice from an eye-specialist is normally needed.

SHORT-SIGHTEDNESS

Some children are short-sighted and will be at a great disadvantage if this is not recognized and treated early. Signs of it are:
- Peering at faces, pictures or books.
- Unawareness of things happening further away from them (babies may take some months to develop this awareness).
- Difficulty reading the blackboard at school.
- Inability to recognize people at a distance.
- Behaviour problems at school (though this may have other causes).

FEBRILE CONVULSIONS

See *Epilepsy* for other types of convulsion.

What are they?

These are a series of sudden jerky movements of arms and legs with a loss of consciousness lasting for 1–2 minutes or longer, in a small child who has a high temperature. They are quite common under the age of 2–3 years, but children usually grow out of them after that, though some may be susceptible to the age of 5 or 6. Febrile convulsions are caused by an excessive rise in temperature.

What to do if your child has one

1 The priority is to **get the temperature down**.
- Strip the child naked, and lie him down on his tummy, face to one side.
- Using a sponge or flannel, wet him *all over* with tepid water: the evaporation of the water cools the body. A gentle fan or the breeze from an open window will help. Keep sponging till the temperature comes down. As it does so, the fit will stop.
2 Then, keep the temperature down:
- Give aspirin or paracetamol 4–6 hourly.

- Do *not* dress the child warmly even if he complains of feeling cold or shivering. A very hot forehead indicates the need for further cooling.
- If this is the first convulsion, take the child to the nearest hospital at once for an examination. In any case, a doctor should see the child to ensure that there is no infection that needs treatment.

3 If the child has more than 2 febrile convulsions he may need to be on a small regular dose of tablets to control this (anti-convulsants) and have check-ups from time to time. Even then it is most important to keep the temperature down.

4 If your child has had febrile convulsions previously, ensure that temperatures do not go up too high (above 38.5°C/101°F or so). Sponge with tepid water, if it does, and give 4–6 hourly doses of aspirin or paracetamol when the temperature is above normal.

GERMAN MEASLES

See *Immunizations in children* and *Common childhood illnesses*.

HEARING PROBLEMS

CONGENITAL DEAFNESS

What is it?
Children who are born deaf have a deficiency of the hearing organs. Their deafness may be partial or complete. They may still be able to appreciate vibrations and, of course, they develop the use of their eyes, minds and hands to take in what is going on around them, if encouraged.

What can be done?
The earlier the deafness is recognized, the sooner teaching and encouragement can be started. This is why, in some countries, hearing tests are performed on babies as young as 3 months. Some centres even have a new electronic hearing tester which can be used on new-born babies.

Parents can contribute by noticing whether, for example, the baby reacts to a voice, a banging door or a loud clap behind his head (where you cannot be seen). If you have any doubts, take your baby to the doctor for a full check-up. In many places there are teachers who specialize in teaching deaf children, and the sooner this teaching can start the better.

ACQUIRED DEAFNESS

What is it?
This is deafness which comes about after birth. It can be the result of several things and may be partial or complete.

If caused by wax
The ear needs syringing after 2–3 days of applying warmed olive oil (2 drops 3 times daily) to soften it. Other drops can be bought that 'dissolve' the wax (Cerumol or Exterol, for example), but can do damage if the problem is *not* one of wax.

If caused by infection
Some ear, nose or throat infections cause a collection of fluid, sometimes pus, in the middle ear behind the ear-drum. Antihistamines or decongestants, such as Actifed, taken by mouth, and Ephedrine Nose Drops may help open up the tube between ear and nose (Eustachian tube) to allow the fluid to drain.

Sometimes acute or chronic infections leave sticky 'gluey' fluid in the middle ear. It is best, if you can, to ask a doctor to examine and treat. See also *Earache*, and *Food allergies*.

If caused by a perforated ear-drum: through trauma
The ear-drum may be burst or perforated as a result of something like a cotton wool bud, bead, or pencil being poked into the ear. There is likely to be some pain when it bursts.

Do not try to remove an object yourself: take the child to a hospital or doctor. Avoid swimming or getting water into the ear. Plug the outside gently with some clean cotton wool while you travel to the doctor.

If you cannot get to a doctor quickly, it may be possible to 'float out' the object (an insect, for example) by instilling some olive oil into the ear; or try sucking it out with a straw, getting someone to hold the child and his head firmly while you do it. Any sudden jerk could cause severe trauma and pain. (See also *First aid*.) However, if the deafness and pain persist, the ear should be examined by a doctor.

If caused by a perforated ear-drum: through infection
Perforated ear-drums can happen as a result of a middle ear infection: the pressure behind the drum builds up and eventually bursts it. There will be a build up of pain, then a sudden relief, together with a discharge of pus and blood.

Again, plug with clean cotton wool and see a doctor for treatment. The drum usually heals over if the infection is cleared up; until it is healed, swimming should be avoided.

The ear should be inspected regularly during the healing process, which may take a few weeks.

Other causes of deafness

These tend to be rare and have to be diagnosed by an ear, nose and throat (ENT) specialist. A child who becomes deaf can be at a great disadvantage at school and with his or her friends, and may develop serious behaviour disorders. It's wise, therefore, to seek help sooner rather than later if you have any suspicions of developing deafness.

HINTS FOR GETTING MEDICINES INTO UNWILLING CHILDREN

● Try not to become anxious about it yourself.
● Explain that it will soon make the child feel better.
● Promise a reward such as a sweet or a story if he takes it.
● 'Give' a dose to a doll or Teddy bear, or take a tiny taste yourself.

If these fail:

● The threat of a treat withheld will sometimes help.
● In a small child you may simply have to hold his hands down firmly and spoon the medicine into his mouth, catching what is spat out and popping it straight back in! Some will be swallowed.

IMMUNIZATIONS IN CHILDREN

Natural immunity

During the first 2–3 months of life a baby is protected against some infections by natural substances called 'antibodies' inherited from the mother through the placenta. Some protection is also given through breast milk. This natural or 'passive' immunity is gradually lost, and must be replaced by the infant's own active resistance to infection.

'Active' immunity or immunization

Our bodies have a very good, though not foolproof, mechanism for developing this resistance. As we meet up with bacteria and viruses in daily living, the white cells in our blood are stimulated to develop specific antibodies which will fight the particular infection. After the first or second occasion of meeting a particular infection, the body will store a small number of these antibodies, and will quickly be able to produce more of the same antibodies to fight that infection another time. This is the basis for vaccination. A child can develop resistance to some serious illnesses by being vaccinated, that is, given very small repeated doses of the modified infection, sufficient to stimulate the production of antibodies, but not to cause the illness.

RECOMMENDED IMMUNIZATION SCHEDULE FOR CHILDREN

These are the vaccinations recommended for small children, and the ages at which they are usually given. The vaccinations may cause a slight fever, or swelling at the site of the injection, but this reaction is far less serious than the illnesses themselves, all of which can kill, or cause serious problems. (See *Whooping cough*.)

	At about 3 months	At about 4 months	At about 5 – 6 months	At 11 – 13 months	At 3 – 5 years (pre-school)
Triple Vaccine (DPT): diphtheria, pertussis (whooping cough), tetanus (Given as one injection or separately.)	FIRST DOSE	SECOND DOSE	THIRD DOSE		BOOSTER
Poliomyelitis (infantile paralysis)	FIRST DOSE	SECOND DOSE	THIRD DOSE		BOOSTER
Measles				One injection only	

COMMON CHILDHOOD ILLNESSES

*See notes on immunization on pages 178–79

Disease	*Whooping cough	Influenza	Meningitis
Organism	A bacterium (Bordetella pertussis)	Several strains of the influenza virus.	May be viral or bacterial
Incubation period	Usually 5–10 days but may be up to 21 days.	1–4 days	2–10 days (bacterial) or variable (viral)
Isolation period (that is: the person is infectious)	Until 2nd or 3rd day of antibiotics.	During acute illness	Strict isolation for duration of illness if of the bacterial variety.
Symptoms	Starts like a cold with runny nose, fever and a cough. 'Whoop' may begin later. The child will have spasms of coughing without stopping between for breath till he coughs up sticky plug of mucus. Then as he breathes in, the air rushes in with a whooping sound. While coughing, face and lips may become blue. The spasms of coughing and the 'whoop' may also lead to vomiting.	Fever, signs of a cold and sore throat, general aches and pains, especially back and legs, sometimes shivering attacks followed by sweating. Usually this stage lasts 3–4 days, then gradually becomes less acute. Usually well in 1–2 weeks. Some people also have headache, vomiting and diarrhoea.	Severe headache, neck stiffness and dislike of light. Fever and increasing drowsiness. High-pitched crying from a baby. Should be seen as soon as possible by a doctor.

COMMON CHILDHOOD ILLNESSES

Disease	*Whooping cough	Influenza	Meningitis
Treatment	Antibiotics (Penicillin, Erythromycin) given in the first week of the illness will modify it and make the child less contagious, but will not affect the length of time the child continues to cough which may be at least 6 weeks. Cough mixture (Actifed compound linctus or Codeine cough linctus) or Eumydrin drops may help stop the vomiting. There is little you can do to help during a coughing spasm. Sit the child up, and remember that the spasm will pass.	Paracetamol (*not* aspirin) every 4–6 hours. Plenty of fluids. Food as desired: appetite will return gradually.	Get immediate medical help. The child (or adult) needs to be in hospital for investigation and treatment.
Complications	Babies under 1 year are at the greatest risk; risks become smaller the older the child.	Occasionally chest infections such as pneumonia. If there is a chesty cough with	See page 127 for details.

COMMON CHILDHOOD ILLNESSES

Disease	*Whooping cough	Influenza	
Complications	Complications include: lung damage, chest infections, including pneumonia, brain damage. Greater risk from illness than from vaccine. **Therefore vaccinate unless specifically told otherwise.** (See also page 190.)	yellow or green phlegm, treat with course of antibiotics.	

Disease	*Diphtheria	*Polio	Mumps
Organism	A bacterium (c. diphtheriae)	Poliomyelitis virus	A virus
Incubation period	2–5 days	7–21 days	Usually 18–21 days
Isolation period (that is: the person is infectious)	Strict isolation until all tests are negative.	Until end of feverish period. Wash hands after touching child.	For 3 weeks from onset of illness.
Symptoms	*Severe* illness with temperature, headache and sore throat.	Starts with the symptoms of a cold, fever, vomiting and sore muscles.	Fever, pain on swallowing and opening mouth. Swelling shows below and in

COMMON CHILDHOOD ILLNESSES

Disease	*Diphtheria	*Polio	Mumps
Symptoms	There may be a yellow-grey membrane coating the back of the throat, sometimes also on nose and lips. Glands become swollen and breath smells bad; there is often difficulty with breathing.	Sometimes when sitting up in bed, the child supports himself on his hands *behind* his back, keeping back stiff.	front of ear, causing child to look like a hamster or goose! May be one-sided only.
Treatment	Isolate. Get *immediate* medical help as there is an anti-toxin and antibiotics that should be given by injection as soon as possible. To prevent: **have your child vaccinated.**	Rest, aspirin or paracetamol regularly to ease the muscle pains. Seek doctor's advice. **The best protection is the polio vaccine: keep it up to date.**	Aspirin or paracetamol for pain and fever. Plenty of fluids. Soft, cool foods (soups, ice cream).
Complications	Difficulty in breathing and other more serious problems. Child should be in hospital.	Paralysis of 1 or more muscles. Medical advice essential, plus rehabilitation after the acute illness is over.	Occasionally affects the testicles, in which case sperm production may go down or stop. Testicle becomes tender and swollen. Treatment: rest, and antibiotics *may* help.

COMMON CHILDHOOD ILLNESSES

Disease	**Tonsillitis**
Organism	A variety of bacteria
Incubation period	2–5 days
Isolation period (that is: the person is infectious)	Not necessary, but avoid breathing and coughing over people.
Symptoms	Feverish illness with enlarged tonsils and glands, sore throat and general aches and pains. Difficulty in swallowing, hoarse voice, bad breath.
Treatment	Antibiotics, bed-rest, fluids and soluble aspirin gargles. (See also page 148.)

COMMON CHILDHOOD ILLNESSES
which cause rashes

Disease	Chicken pox	*German measles	Non-specific fevers
Organism	A virus (Varicella zoster)	The Rubella virus	A virus (Echo and others)
Incubation period	14–21 days	14–21 days	5–10 days
Type of rash	Crops of small, itchy blisters, with clear fluid initially. Become pus-filled, break and crust over.	Very fine pink spots which turn white on pressure. Usually very mild associated symptoms.	Fine pink spots which turn white on pressure. Associated 'cold' symptoms.
Distribution over body	Densest on the body, spreading to limbs and face.	Starts behind the ears and spreads to body and limbs.	Face and body.
Duration of rash	10–12 days	2–3 days	2–3 days
Infective period	5 days before rash till 6 days after last crop of blisters or till blisters are crusted over and dry.	7 days before rash to 4 days after disappearance.	7 days before rash to 4 days after disappearance.
Symptoms other than rash	Fever, sore throat, itching blisters, abdominal pain.	Usually minimal. Headache, sore throat, fever, mild conjunctivitis. Some glands up.	Mild to severe catarrh, sore throat, diarrhoea, conjunctivitis.

COMMON CHILDHOOD ILLNESSES
which cause rashes

Disease	Chicken pox	*German measles	Non-specific fevers
Treatment	Daily bathing with mild antiseptic or salt water. Calamine lotion or Piriton may help the itching. Antibiotic eye ointment if blister appears in eye. Paracetamol for fever.	None. Aspirin or paracetamol if feverish and miserable. Keep away from, and warn, pregnant mothers.	None apart from aspirin, paracetamol and cough mixture as necessary.
Complications	Secondary bacterial infection of blisters, skin, and of the breathing tubes. Treat with Antibiotics; see doctor if child becomes worse.	Rare in children. Adults may develop joint-pains and swelling. Abnormalities of the unborn affected child.	Rare.

Disease	Scarlet fever	*Measles
Organism	A bacterium (streptococcus)	The measles virus
Incubation period	1–3 days	12–21 days
Type of rash	Small red or pink spots which turn white on pressure. Coated tongue with prominent tastebuds:	Initially red or pink spots which run together so that the skin appears blotchy all over. May stain the skin.

COMMON CHILDHOOD ILLNESSES
which cause rashes

Disease	Scarlet fever	*Measles
	'strawberry tongue'. Flushed face, white around mouth.	Spots appear on the 4th day of the illness.
Distribution over body	Body and limbs. Flushed face. Sometimes red patches appear on legs.	First appears behind the ears and in the hairline, then spreads to face and body. For first 2–3 days, white patches (Koplic spots) inside cheeks.
Duration of rash	4–5 days	7–10 days
Infective period	Until 1–2 days after antibiotics commence.	For 14 days from onset.
Symptoms other than rash	Acute onset of illness, sore throat, fever, nausea, vomiting, headache.	Acute onset of fever, catarrh, conjunctivitis; by day 2, eyes become very sensitive to light, hoarse voice, cough.
Treatment	Penicillin or Erythromycin (that is: antibiotic treatment since this is a bacterial infection)	Isolation, aspirin or paracetamol, cough linctus, darkened room. Antibiotic eye ointment if discharge develops.

COMMON CHILDHOOD ILLNESSES
which cause rashes

Disease	Scarlet fever	*Measles
Complications	Ear infection, sinusitis. *Occasionally* more serious. Change antibiotics if they are not controlling complications. See doctor if child becomes rapidly worse.	Ear infections, chest infection, eye complications, convulsions. See a doctor if child is developing any of these or becoming worse rapidly. In a malnourished child, measles can be very severe.

INFLUENZA
See *Common childhood illnesses*.

MEASLES
See *Immunizations in children*.

MENINGITIS
See *Common childhood illnesses*.

MUMPS
See *Common childhood illnesses*.

NAPPY RASH
See *Common problems in the first few weeks*, section 7.

NON-SPECIFIC FEVERS
See *Common childhood illnesses*.

POLIO
See *Immunizations in children*.

RUBELLA
See *Immunizations in children*.

SCARLET FEVER
See *Common childhood illnesses*.

TEMPER TANTRUMS

What are they?
These are expressions of extreme frustration, and it is the frustration that needs to be dealt with.

What to do during a tantrum
● Allow the child to express his frustration fully. He or she will stop when exhausted, or if a breath-holding attack occurs.
● Do not make a big fuss about it, either in terms of anger or a great deal of 'cuddling'.
● Do not give in to the demand that led to the tantrum in order to keep the peace. A child will always know how to 'twist your arm' another time!
● Try not to let the child see how upset you become if the tantrum happens in a public place; you should, of course, make it clear that you are angry (if you are) but do this later when talking with him or her about it.

What to do after a tantrum
Do talk with your child about why you do not give in, or allow him or her to have what was wanted. If possible, let the child explain the frustration. Even small children respond eventually to explanation and firmness. You may have to resort to some form of disciplinary action if nothing else works.

Preventive action
Distract the child's attention to something else as soon as a temper tantrum threatens.

UNDESCENDED TESTICLES

How does this happen?
The testicles develop inside the abdomen and gradually work their way out and down into the scrotum through the groin (or inguinal canal). At birth the testicles of most baby boys are already there or almost there, but they can be readily pulled back up into the inguinal canal (a reflex reaction to cold or touch). The muscle then relaxes and allows the testicles to descend again into the scrotum where they can be kept cooler than body temperature. In children with undescended testicles, they are usually still in the abdomen or in the canal. Often, they will descend of their own accord within the first few years of life.

What is the treatment?

Surgery may be necessary to bring down and fix the testicle(s) in the scrotum. This is usually done between the ages of 3-5. If it is not done within a year or two of this, there may be damage to the sperm, or sperm production, by the heat of the body.

WHEEZING

What is it?

Children who wheeze breathe with difficulty, producing a hoarse whistling sound. Some get a certain amount of wheezing when they have a chest infection. This is sometimes known as a 'wheezy bronchitis'. Usually this is not the same as an attack of asthma, nor do babies who have this necessarily become asthmatics.

In more serious cases

If a baby or a toddler has wheezing and a chest infection, watch the chest for:
● A number of breaths per minute (respiratory rate) of over 60.
● Ribs becoming clearly marked with the spaces between them drawn in and the abdomen protruding with each breath.

Treatment

If these signs develop, or there is any difficulty in breathing, the child must be taken to hospital as soon as possible. He may need treatment in a steam tent and receive oxygen; he may need other medications. You can help initially by taking him into a room which is as steamed up as possible (run the hot tap or shower, or boil pans or kettles of water).

WHOOPING COUGH

See also *Immunizations in children*.

The illness itself is very dangerous in children under 6 months, slightly less so from 6-12 months, and although it may be severe and quite a nuisance in older children, there is less risk of long-term complications.

Vaccination

There has been much discussion about the risks of giving the vaccination, which has led to many parents not having their child vaccinated. The consequences are that there seem to be more epidemics of whooping cough occurring and many more children will, once again, suffer the long-term complications of the disease. The risk of brain damage after the vaccination is minimal, but it should not be given to a baby who has had convulsions, or if there is a

history of epilepsy in the
immediate family.

What is the treatment?

Those who have not been
vaccinated should be treated
with Penicillin, Erythromycin, or
Septrin (see *Common drugs*,
section 8) as soon as possible
if they develop a cough after
contact with whooping cough,
or if there is an epidemic.
Antibiotics will prevent others
being infected. However, after
the first week, antibiotics make
no difference to the length of
time the child continues to
cough after the initial infection:
this may be 6 weeks or longer
in any case. If the child (or
you) is becoming exhausted by
the coughing, then regular
doses of cough mixture may
help to control it to some
extent. A drink and perhaps
some food after a spasm of
coughing will help to combat
the exhaustion.

During a spasm of coughing

● Ensure the mouth is empty.
● Sit or prop the child up.
● Stay with him during a
  spasm.
● Keep a bowl or bucket
  handy in case he vomits.
● Comfort him with a cuddle
  after the spasm has ended.
● Give him a drink when the
  coughing has stopped.

6. COMMON TROPICAL PROBLEMS

AMOEBIASIS

What is it?
This is a condition caused by an amoeba known as Entamoeba histolytica. The infection is acquired by eating or drinking anything that has been contaminated by the waste matter (excreta) of an already infected person.

What are the symptoms?
The person usually suffers from diarrhoea mixed with mucus and blood and from abdominal pains. In more severe and prolonged cases it can cause a liver abscess.

How is it diagnosed?
The stools of the patient need to be examined under a microscope.

Treatment
Metronidazole (Flagyl) 400mg 3 times daily for 7 days is the usual treatment. (Sometimes higher doses are needed.) Follow-up stool tests should be done after treatment on 3 stools on different days. The side-effects of this drug are:
● A metallic taste in the mouth.
● Nausea and loss of appetite.
● If alcohol is drunk with this, severe nausea and perhaps vomiting.

BILHARZIA

What is it?
This is an infection by blood flukes (parasitic flatworms) of 3 different types, 2 of which inhabit the veins of the gut, while the third inhabits the veins of the bladder. The larvae of the flukes must live part of their life-cycle in fresh-water snails, and infect humans by 'boring' through the skin as they drink, wade or swim in infected water. The young flukes develop into adults in the human blood system, and the eggs pass out in human excreta.

Where does it occur?
One 'gut fluke' and one 'bladder fluke' occur in Africa (mainly East) and the Middle East, and also in parts of South America. The other 'gut fluke' lives in parts of China, the Philippines, Sulawesi and some parts of Japan.

Prevention
● Keep out of water that might be infected.

- Boil all drinking water from such sources.
- Eliminate, or at least reduce, the snail population.
- Educate people *not* to use the area near water sources as a toilet.
- Treat infected individuals.

Symptoms

- 'Swimmer's itch', a local irritation where the developing flukes have penetrated the skin.
- Blood in stools or urine.
- Unexplained prolonged fever, malaise, or weight-loss.

Treatment

Permanent or fatal damage can be done when infected over a long period of time, so diagnosis and treatment by a hospital with laboratory facilities is important. Urine and stool tests may be sufficient to diagnose the illness, but more sophisticated tests (including a blood test) are sometimes necessary.

CHOLERA

What is it?

It is an infection with the cholera organism, which causes inflammation of the whole of the small intestine. It tends to occur in epidemics, and is common in Asia, the Middle East and Africa.

How is it spread?

It is spread by the eating or drinking of food or water contaminated by infected stools (faeces). The incubation period is 1–3 days.

What are the symptoms?

- Profuse watery diarrhoea, of sudden onset and with no pain. The watery stools are sometimes described as like 'rice-water' in appearance.
- Vomiting may also occur.
- Muscle cramps; weakness and thirst.
- Increasing tendency to 'dry out' (dehydration), if the fluid loss is not rapidly replaced. It is this that can kill the patient.

What is the treatment?

Fluid replacement is the most important treatment; if the person is vomiting he will need to be admitted to hospital for fluid replacement through a vein (intravenous). It can be started using the Oral Rehydration Solution (see *Diarrhoea*) given in small sips more or less continuously, until medical help is available.
NOTE
Children become dehydrated even more quickly than adults, and they will need prompt and continuous fluid replacement, by teaspoon if necessary. Seek medical help quickly.

How can it be prevented?

- Food and water hygiene.

- Cholera vaccination (see *Immunization*, section 4.1).
- Tetracycline given to people close to the infected person (250mg 6-hourly for 7 days) is effective in preventing further spread within a household.

CUTANEOUS LARVA MIGRANS

What is it?
It is a winding, threadlike trail of inflammation in the skin (also called 'creeping eruptions') caused by the larvae of worms that do not usually infest man: the dog or cat hookworm, for example. The larva burrows into the skin from infected soil, slowly moving forwards under the skin, leaving an inflamed trail behind it and causing severe itching and irritation.

How can it be treated?
A 10% suspension of thiabendazole may be applied to the inflamed area 4 times a day for 7 – 10 days.

DENGUE FEVER

What is it?
It is an acute infection (also called 'break-bone fever') caused by a virus and transmitted from person to person by the bite of certain mosquitoes.

Where does it occur?
South-east Asia, but also most tropical and sub-tropical regions.

What effect does it have?
It causes a sudden onset of fever, lasting about 7 days, with severe pains in the joints and back, headache and measles-like rash.

How serious is it?
The disease is not usually dangerous and is usually mild in children.

What is the treatment?
Treat as for a fever and take aspirin or paracetamol (2 tablets 4-hourly) for pain. Unfortunately, as it is caused by a virus, antibiotics will not be effective.

FILARIASIS
See also *Onchocerciasis* and *Loa Loa* for different forms of microfilariae.

What is it?
It is a group of illnesses caused by several different minute worms known as 'microfilariae'. These are carried by various types of mosquito (the Aëdes, Culex and Anopholes) and injected into the bloodstream when a person is bitten. The microfilariae develop in the bloodstream and eventually 'lodge' in the lymphatic

system, including the lymph nodes.

What is the incubation period?
Two to 8 months or more.

What are the symptoms and signs?
Chills, fever, headache and general malaise. The fever in some types typically occurs at nights. Eventually the microfilariae, if present in large numbers, will 'clog up' the lymph nodes, leading to a swelling of the glands and the tissues usually drained through those glands. This may cause elephantiasis of the leg, with swollen, enlarged glands in the groin.

What is the treatment?
Usually 2–4 weeks of drug treatment under medical supervision; occasionally, surgery to relieve the swellings.

How can it be prevented?
Avoid the mosquito! (See also section on *Malaria*.)
● Prevent breeding by clearing the breeding sites: stagnant pools or collections of water in tins and so on.
● Kill the mosquitoes with sprays.
● Avoid being bitten by wearing long sleeves and trousers, using insect repel -lants and mosquito nets.

GIARDIASIS

What is the cause?
Giardiasis is caused by the parasite giardia lamblia, which is taken into the body through food and water contaminated by infected human excreta. It usually causes diarrhoea, but often causes only mild indigestion, abdominal discomfort and wind. If the parasite gets into the cells lining the gut it can cause more general symptoms of tiredness or general malaise which may drag on and become a chronic illness.

What is the treatment?
Metronidazole (Flagyl) in large doses (such as 2000mg daily for 3 days, repeated 1 week later). It should be supervised by a doctor. It is likely to make you feel very nauseated especially if taken with alcohol! Follow-up stool tests should be done on 3 different occasions after treatment.

GUINEA WORM

What is it?
This is a disease caused by the presence of the guinea worm in the tissues just under the skin. It occurs in India, Pakistan, the Middle East, tropical Africa, certain West Indian islands and the Guineas. It is caught by drinking water infested with the

larvae of the Guinea worm. These develop and eventually reach the tissues below the skin as adult worms.

What are the symptoms and signs?
Intensely itchy swelling which ulcerates. Through this ulcer the female worm discharges the larvae (which enter water when the infected person walks or swims in a stream or pond).

What is the treatment?
- Niridazole or Thiabendazole may kill the worm. Ask a doctor for advice as this may cause more problems!
- Gradual extraction by winding the worm round a twig or similar over 10 days.
- Antiseptic soaks (Dettol, TCP or similar) and creams to prevent bacterial infection (Savlon cream), antibiotics if the ulcer becomes infected. It is best, if possible, to have medical supervision.

How can it be prevented?
- Never drink unfiltered, unboiled water from uncovered ponds or from streams or rivers where people may have walked or swum.
- Promote any local efforts to cover water holes and ponds used to collect drinking water, and discourage people from walking into these.

HEAT PROBLEMS

There are several degrees of reaction to excessive heat, heat stroke being the severest. Most people experience some loss of energy in a hot climate, especially if it is humid. They find themselves less active both mentally and physically (some experience this more than others). It does not have to be direct sunlight: it is the 'heat load' that is important.

MILD HEAT FATIGUE

What are the symptoms?
- Loss of energy.
- Loss of efficiency, mental and physical.

What is the treatment?
- Don't go out, or stay out, in the sun for longer than necessary.
- Cool showers will help.
- Drink enough fluids and add extra salt to your food to replace what you lose in sweat. An adult should need a *minimum* of 3 litres in 24 hours, more if you are sweating; a small child (1–5 years) needs a *minimum* of 1 litre; a baby needs ½–1 litre. (Beware of over-loading babies and small children with salt: see the oral rehydration solution recommended under *Diarrhoea*.)

PRICKLY HEAT

What is it?
A fine red rash of very tiny blisters on any part of the body, especially those covered by non-absorbent material made of nylon or other man-made fibres. There is itching or irritation. It is common in both children and adults.

What is the treatment?
- Always wear cotton clothing, especially underwear.
- Cool showers, drinks, and so on to cool down and keep cool.
- Calamine lotion or other soothing creams applied to the rash if necessary, but it is best if the air can be allowed to get at the area.

HEAT CRAMPS

What are they?
These are painful muscular cramps or spasms in legs, arms or wall of the abdomen, and are the result of not eating enough salt to replace what you lose in sweat.

What is the treatment?
Add extra salt to your food or drink. Take salt tablets if you do not like salt in your food but no more than 1 – 2 salt tablets a day, however, unless otherwise advised by a doctor.

NOTE
Small children should be given the properly made-up oral rehydration solution. (See section on *Diarrhoea*.)

HEAT EXHAUSTION

What are the causes?
This is due, again, to not drinking enough water and not eating enough salt to replace what you are losing in sweat and other fluids.

What are the symptoms?
Headache, dizziness, nausea, feeling faint, profuse sweating with a cool, moist skin. The person will be *pale* and may not feel thirsty.

What is the treatment?
- Cool down: sit in the shade, remove outer clothing and increase the air flow with a fan or ask a friend to do this for you.
- Lie down flat with legs raised above head level until you feel better.
- Drink 3 – 5 litres of water with salt added (½ teaspoon salt to 1 litre of water) over the next 12 – 24 hours. (See section on *Diarrhoea* for correct oral rehydration solution.) Diluted Coca Cola (½:½) will help at first if you are travelling or in a situation where you cannot make up the mixture.

● If vomiting is a problem, drink 2–3 sips of oral rehydration solution every 10 minutes: some will stay down. If you are feeling faint, vomiting, or not passing much water, seek medical help, but get on with the drinking!

'HEAT STROKE'

What is it?

This is much more serious than any of the above and needs medical care. The heat-regulating mechanism ceases to function and the temperature rises to dangerous levels. So, while someone arranges for medical help, or while you are taking the person to hospital, **get the temperature down**.

'Heat stroke' can occur with malaria or other feverish illnesses where shivering has led to clothing being piled on, or as a result of exposure to intense sun and heat.

What are the symptoms?

● Headache, dizziness, vomiting.
● Very hot, dry skin: the face and body will be red with no sweating and a high temperature (may go above 40.5°C/105°F).
● In severe cases, or if the temperature is not brought down quickly, delirium, loss of consciousness, and convulsions.

What is the treatment?

The aim is to get the temperature down quickly.

● Get the person into a shaded place with a good through-draught of air.
● Strip him or her naked.
● If a bath is available, immerse the whole body in cold water, adding ice where possible.

If there is no bath, sprinkle the whole body continuously with cold water from a watering can or similar, or just pour it over the body. Increase the draught by using a fan or flapping a large sheet or similar over the body.

Otherwise wring out a sheet or tablecloth in any available cold water (river, pond) and wrap the person in this, repeating the process as the sheet becomes warm. Keep the draught going. Use pond water even in areas where there is a risk of bilharzia, if there is no other water available: the bilharzia can be treated later.

Keep this up until the temperature has come down to below 38.5°C/101°F and watch for further rises over the the next 12–24 hours.

● Get medical help as soon as possible.

HEPATITIS

What is it?
This is an inflammation of the liver caused by at least 2 types of viruses, commonly referred to as hepatitis A and hepatitis B. They both tend to cause a yellow discolouration of the skin and whites of the eyes called jaundice, which can also be caused by other illnesses. Gamma-globulin, which is not a vaccine, gives useful protection against hepatitis A and there is a vaccine against hepatitis B now available.

HEPATITIS A
This is the common variety, also known as infectious hepatitis, particularly widespread in tropical countries.

How is it passed on?
Contamination of food and water with human faeces or close contact with someone who has hepatitis.

How can it be prevented?
- Boil all drinking water for 5 minutes.
- Always wash your hands after going to the toilet.
- Wash your hands before preparing or eating food.
- Wash all vegetables and fruit to be eaten raw in boiled or chlorinated water. Beware of salads and fresh fruit in hotels and road-side cafés: they may have been washed in contaminated water or prepared by contaminated hands! Beware also of ice cream and ice cubes.
- Keep all foods covered, and where possible, do not eat food that has had flies on it.
- Cook all sea-foods and meat thoroughly.
- Have regular 6-monthly gamma-globulin injections, if available, or have a booster if you have a known contact with hepatitis or a local epidemic.

What are the symptoms?
The incubation period is 3–5 weeks. It develops gradually, with vague malaise, abnormal tiredness, lack of appetite, head and body aches, low-grade fever, nausea, vomiting and loss of weight. There is also pain in the upper part of the abdomen, on the right under the ribs, yellow discolouration of the skin and whites of the eyes, dark tea-coloured urine and pale stools. Depression often develops.

What is the treatment?
There is no specific treatment that will cure, but you should see a doctor who can make the diagnosis and monitor your progress. Some treatment may be necessary, depending on the severity of the illness. The basic treatment is rest and a special diet.

Special diet

The liver is unable to do its usual efficient job of breaking down complicated foods into simple usable components, so a high carbohydrate (starches, grains, cereals, fruit, vegetables) and low protein (though some fish, chicken or similar should be taken), low fat diet is advisable (and generally more acceptable anyway, when feeling nauseated). **Drink no alcohol** (some advise none for 6–12 months after an attack of hepatitis).

Rest

Physical rest is essential; not resting will only prolong the recovery.

Hygiene

Scrupulous personal hygiene, as urine and stools are a source of infection to others.

Depression

If you become depressed, remember that this *will* clear up as the illness clears, but that the illness will usually last for at least a month, and physical and mental tiredness may last for several months after an attack. Accept some limitations during this recovery time, aiming at a gradual resumption of normal physical activities. Gradually increasing exercise, starting slowly and building up each week, will help.

Is there a vaccine against hepatitis A?

There is no 'active' immunization as yet, that is, one that will stimulate your own antibody production. Work is in progress on developing one. However, there is 'passive' immunization with gamma-globulin, which will give you significant, though not 100%, protection for 4–6 months. As its effect wears off, theoretically, you develop your own immunity, as you meet up with the virus while partially protected. It probably gives little protection against hepatitis B.

Can you get it twice?

Once you have had hepatitis A, or have had contact with it, your own immune system develops antibodies against it. Then you should not get hepatitis again and gamma-globulin is not needed. Quite a significant number of people are already immune although they have not had the illness.

Should children have gamma-globulin?

Yes, in appropriately reduced doses, if they are not already immune. Hepatitis A in children is usually mild, however. Gamma-globulin can inhibit the immune response, so babies who are receiving their triple vaccine (diphtheria, whooping cough and tetanus), and their polio and measles vaccines (during their first year), should not be given it.

Should you insist on having gamma-globulin?

Your doctor may tell you that this is of little use. Do insist, however, if you are not already immune, if you are travelling to or living in an area where there is a high incidence of hepatitis A. Some protection is always better than none. Even if it does not give 100% protection it will modify the severity of the illness if you should develop it. Hepatitis can be such a long drawn-out illness that it is devastating to get it.

HEPATITIS B

This condition, also known as serum hepatitis, is much rarer than A, thankfully, as it can be quite severe.

How is it passed on?

'Blood-to-blood' on contaminated needles and syringes, acupuncture needles, tattooing, and ear piercing; through cuts and abrasions and possibly through blood-sucking insects.

How can it be prevented?

● Avoid contact with anything contaminated!
● The virus can be transmitted through body secretions such as saliva, so *close* physical contact (kissing, sexual intercourse), should be avoided with someone

who has this.

● Hepatitis B vaccine is available and is recommended for those at special risk.

What are the symptoms?

The incubation period is 6 weeks to 5 months. The symptoms are the same as for Infectious Hepatitis.

What is the treatment?

As for Infectious Hepatitis. Only blood tests will be able to differentiate between A and B types, and you will need to be under the care of a doctor.

LASSA FEVER

What is it?

This is one of several viral illnesses which may be caught from animals who usually harbour the virus. The Lassa fever virus is carried by certain rats in West Africa who excrete the virus in their urine. Marburg virus disease is caused by a virus carried by the African green monkey. The Ebola virus is also thought to be carried by an animal. All these may cause serious illness, even death, and skilled care in hospital is necessary.

What are the Lassa fever symptoms?

Those of an ordinary influenza type of illness with a very

sudden and severe deterioration after 3–6 days. Any such deterioration in any illness should prompt you to call for medical help as quickly as possible.

LEECHES

What are they?
These are aquatic worms that suck blood. They may be troublesome near streams or in damp forests, when they may find their way through laced boots or shoes. Their bites are painless, but may bleed or turn septic. Leeches should not be dragged off the skin, because of the increased danger of infection if their 'suction apparatus' is left behind. If the leech is touched with a lighted cigarette, or covered with salt, lemon juice or vinegar, it will drop off and the bite can then be cleaned with antiseptic.

LEISHMANIASIS

What is it?
This is a group of illnesses caused by a parasite called Leishmania and transmitted by the bite of the sandfly 'Phlebotomus'. Depending on the form of the parasite, the illness may show itself as kala-azar, oriental sore, American leishmaniasis, or diffuse cutaneous leishmaniasis.

What are the symptoms and signs?

KALA-AZAR
● A long-term chronic illness with fever occurring irregularly.
● It occurs in India, China, Russia, Africa, Mediterranean basin, South and Central America.

ORIENTAL SORE
● One or more ulcers persisting for 2–18 months and eventually healing spontaneously.
● It occurs in India, China, the Mediterranean and North Africa.

AMERICAN LEISHMANIASIS
● A persisting ulceration of the nose and back of the mouth. Does not heal spontaneously and can be very disfiguring.
● It occurs in Mexico, Central and South America.

DIFFUSE CUTANEOUS LEISHMANIASIS
● Causes widespread skin lesions resembling leprosy.
● It occurs in South America and Ethiopia.

What is the treatment?
All types need drug treatment under medical supervision.

How can it be prevented?
● Avoid the sandfly!

- Promote any local efforts to clear breeding sites, and kill off the sandfly.

LEPROSY

What is it?
It is an infection caused by the Mycobacterium leprae affecting the skin and nerves. It is found all over the world where poverty and overcrowding encourage it to spread from person to person. It is not especially associated with warm climates. The World Health Organization estimated that there were at least 15 million people with leprosy in 1980. Only about 2.5 million of these have ever been treated.

How is it spread?
It may be spread by prolonged body contact, but it may also be passed on when a person inhales the thousands of bacteria that an infected person expels when he sneezes. The ulcers formed also shed bacteria. Millions of people are exposed to possible infection, but there seems to be some individual sensitivity that leads only certain people to develop it.

What are the symptoms of an initial infection?
The symptoms are usually so minor that they go unnoticed. Many never develop any obvious disease, recovering completely from the infection, and perhaps developing some immunity, rather like the result of a vaccination. Others will develop an obvious clinical disease, probably after many years, and the outcome will depend on the person's resistance to the infection.

What are the later problems?
The bacteria mainly attack the nerves, the skin and the nose, but also many other organs. The most obvious problems that develop are therefore:

- Loss of sensation: fingers and toes are not able to feel when they have been injured or burned. The injuries often become infected and tissue may be destroyed if not properly treated and further injury avoided. The person with leprosy has to learn to do a thorough daily check for any injuries, and shoes have to be very specially made so that they cannot rub anywhere and cause ulcers.
- Patches on the skin which are discoloured or have no colour, with loss of sensation. The skin may also become thickened or ulcerated and scarred, often causing disfigurement, especially of the face.

Can it be treated?
Yes, it can be treated very successfully, especially if

found in the early stages before any disfigurement or loss of tissue (particularly of fingers and toes) has occurred. But it takes a great deal of commitment and money, both by health personnel and programme planners, to set up wide-scale screening programmes. A great deal of re-education is also needed world-wide to teach people that

- Leprosy is treatable.
- Leprosy is preventable.
- Leprosy sufferers need not be isolated away from other people; they can live in their own communities and be treated and receive follow-up there. Once they have received a certain amount of treatment they are no longer infectious.

LIVER FLUKES

What are they?
There are several varieties of fluke (parasitic flatworm) that infest the liver. They are caught by eating raw or partly cooked fish, because the larvae (called Cercariae) all inhabit a variety of fish. The eggs develop in fresh water snails of a certain type (operculated) and pass out into the water where they enter into susceptible fish.

What are the symptoms?
These depend on the number of flukes infesting the liver but the main problem is recurrent bouts of jaundice (yellow discolouration of the skin) with other signs of an inflammation of the liver (there may be fever, and tenderness in the right upper part of the abdomen).

How can they be avoided?
Avoid eating raw or partly cooked fish.

How is it treated?
With a drug called praziquantel.

LOA LOA

What is it?
It is a form of filariasis caused by Loa Loa and transmitted by the bite of the Chrysops fly. It occurs in Central and West Africa.

What are the symptoms and signs?
Localized transient swellings (Calabar swellings) under the skin caused by the migration of the worms through the tissues and the release of irritants. They may also migrate across the eye.

How is it treated?
Usually 2–4 weeks of drug treatment under medical supervision; occasionally, surgery to relieve the swellings if they persist.

How can it be prevented?
Avoid the Chrysops fly!

MALARIA

What is it?
It is one of the most widespread of all tropical diseases, causing many deaths and much ill-health. It occurs in most of the tropical and sub-tropical parts of the world. It is caused by infection with an organism collectively known as Plasmodium, but with 4 species causing human illness:
- P. falciparum (malignant tertian malaria or cerebral malaria).
- P. vivax.
- P. ovale.
- P. malariae.

How is it caught?
The plasmodium is carried by the female Anopholes mosquito and injected together with the saliva when the mosquito bites a human being. Thousands of organisms may be injected in a single bite. The organisms enter the liver through the bloodstream and multiply there for varying periods of time until they are released back into the bloodstream to invade the red blood cells.

Inside the red cells they divide and multiply until they rupture the cell, again releasing thousands of organisms into the circulation.

It is at this stage that the infected person develops the typical fever of malaria. Many of these new organisms will re-invade other red cells, and after varying periods of delay, cause further attacks of fever.

What are the symptoms?
If you have been taking anti-malarials, the following description may not apply, or you may have a similar but not so severe attack. A classical attack of malaria, of whatever type, is as follows:
- A cold stage: severe shivering or uncontrollable shaking and shivering (rigor), more severe than the chills people get with, for example, influenza. The temperature starts going up quickly.
- A hot stage: the person is flushed and very hot, with a severe headache and fast pulse rate. The temperature stays high for a few hours.
- A sweating stage: the person starts sweating profusely as the temperature drops down back to normal or near-normal.

P. vivax typically causes this sort of an attack; P. falciparum may not cause the rigor, but is more likely to cause very high temperature rises and delirium. This is the malignant or dangerous variety and may cause death if not treated quickly.

All forms of malaria may cause recurring attacks of fever, with varying intervals free. In untreated cases the attacks may continue for years: up to 1 year in the case of P. falciparum (unless re-infection occurs) and up to 30 years with P. malariae, with the severity of the attacks likely to diminish with time.

In a person who has been taking anti-malarials, the symptoms may include episodes of the following:

● Headaches and general muscle aches and pains.
● Nausea and vomiting.
● Diarrhoea.
● Non-specific general malaise.

How is malaria diagnosed?

If at all possible, a blood test should be done. Blood is spread on a slide and examined under the microscope for the presence of the malaria parasite. This should be done during an attack, if possible, as this is the time the plasmodium is most plentifully present in the circulation.

What is the treatment?

In the absence of a doctor and laboratory facilities, and if the symptoms are not very severe, anti-malarial tablets will help. However, if your area is known to have P. falciparium, especially if it is the resistant

variety, and the attack is severe (with a high temperature, severe headache, vomiting and delirium), medical help must be sought urgently. Otherwise:

● Start taking a full course of Chloroquine or Fansidar (see *Malaria, protection and treatment*, in section 4 for details).
● Keep sipping at cool fluids, even if vomiting occurs.
● Take aspirin or paracetamol 2 tablets 4-hourly (or, for stronger pain-killers, see *Common drugs*, section 8), for the headache and general muscle aches and pains.
● Check the temperature from time to time; if it is above 40°C/104°F, cool the person down with tepid sponging (see *Heat stroke*).

What does 'resistance' mean?

The plasmodium is very 'clever' in that it is able to protect itself against many of the drugs that are used against it, especially if full dosages or courses are not taken. Thus new strains continue to emerge that are 'resistant' to Chloroquine, and more recently, sometimes resistant to Maloprim and Fansidar, and the other anti-malarials.

New drugs are being developed and tried out, and will be increasingly available. However, the World Health

Organization and other concerned bodies are anxious that the newer drugs should not also be improperly used and thereby increase the chances of resistance developing to these as well. Quinine is coming back into use but requires medical supervision.

Malaria and pregnancy
See *Malaria*, section 4 for details, also *Pregnancy*, section 7.

Malaria prophyllaxis
See *Malaria*, section 4 for details.

ONCHOCERCIASIS

What is it?
This disease, also known as 'river blindness', is caused by a minute worm (microfilaria) called Onchocerca volvulus. This is carried by the black fly (Simulium) and occurs in Central and South America, West and Central Africa and Yemen. The illness can take months to develop and may become a chronic condition.

What are the symptoms and signs?
Extreme itching, with a rash (like nettle-rash) in the skin and tissues just below the skin. The microfilariae sometimes get into the eyes and can occasionally be seen

'travelling' across the eye. It is called 'river blindness' because the fly lives along rivers and the infected eye can sometimes become inflamed and blind, but only in cases of heavy infestation.

How is it treated?
Usually 2–4 weeks of drug treatment which must be under medical supervision.

How can it be prevented?
● Avoid being bitten! But the fly is tiny, persistent and difficult to avoid. Insect repellants may help.
● Help any local efforts to kill off the black flies breeding in fast rivers.

RABIES
See section 5.1.

SCRUB TYPHUS
This is common in South-east Asia, Oceania, Northern Australia and South-east Siberia. It is also known as mite typhus and tsutsugamushi fever and is transmitted through the bite of a mite that lives on rodents.

What are the symptoms?
● At the site of the bite, a small swelling forms that ulcerates and forms a 'black eschar' or chronic ulcer.
● 4–14 days later, there is usually fever, general aches

and pains and headache.
- In severe cases, a cough develops, with swollen glands, a rash over body, upper arms and legs and the patient becomes very sensitive to light.

What is the treatment?
In mild cases, treat as for any fever (see *Fever*). In severe cases, the person should be treated in hospital with antibiotics and nursing care.

How can it be prevented?
- Destroy mite-infested areas.
- Spray mite-infested houses with insecticide.
- Wear protective clothing and use insect-repellants.

SPRUE — Tropical

What is it?
This is a condition in which a person develops persistent long-term diarrhoea which can lead on to vitamin deficiencies and anaemia. It is often triggered off by a severe episode of diarrhoea, or several recurrent episodes causing an inflammatory reaction of the lining of the intestines. There is usually an increased loss of fat in the stools which tend to float in the water of the toilet. Any diarrhoea that continues for more than 1 or 2 weeks should be investigated. Treatment will

depend on the findings and diagnosis.

TICK FEVER

What is it?
It is also known as relapsing fever or tick typhus. It is a group of fevers caused by the bites of infected ticks which have fed on the blood of the animals (probably rodents) carrying the organism. The illnesses are usually mild feverish ones, and should be treated as for any fever. (See *Fever*.)

How can it be prevented?
Avoid tick-bites by
- Wearing protective clothing and using insect repellants when camping.
- Regular inspection of pets for ticks.

Louse-borne fever
(also relapsing fever) is carried by the body louse, and causes a similar illness to tick fever.

TUBERCULOSIS

What is it?
TB is a chronic infection of the lungs (usually) or any part of the body, caused by the tubercle bacillus. It is what was once called 'consumption', and is still very widespread in tropical and sub-tropical countries.

How is it caught?

Lung or pulmonary TB is caught by breathing in the tubercle bacillus in tiny droplets of phlegm coughed out by a person who has the active disease.

How can it be prevented?

- BCG Vaccination at birth probably gives life-long immunity to most people.
- BCG Vaccination later if not at birth. The need for this should be checked by a skin-test first: if you have already had contact with the tubercle bacillus and developed immunity, the BCG could give you a severe reaction.
- Avoid close contact with those you know have 'open' TB (that is, they are coughing up bacilli). Not everyone with TB does this, and regular sputum tests are done on those who are having treatment to check if they are. If you have had a BCG however, you are reasonably safe, and there is no need to keep your distance!

What is the treatment?

Injections and medicines, which must be taken regularly and for the full course recommended by the doctor, anything from 6–24 months. **If the treatment is stopped too soon the bacilli become resistant and may cause a more severe illness which is very difficult to treat.**

Other kinds of TB

The TB infection may be focused in the glands or bone, or in any organ, having been carried through the blood-stream to that point. The treatment for all types of TB is the same.

Diet

As with any infection, a good, balanced diet, with adequate rest and exercise will help.

TYPHOID

What is it?

Typhoid is a serious feverish illness caused by the typhoid bacteria, which infects primarily the gut, causing abdominal pain and diarrhoea initially, but sometimes constipation later. Paratyphoid is a milder illness caused by related organisms.

How is it caught?

By contamination of food or water by human faeces.

How can it be prevented?

- By ensuring your own hands or those of anyone preparing your food are carefully washed after using the toilet and before handling any food.
- Boil all drinking water for at least 5 minutes.

- Keep all food covered against flies.
- Keep up *yearly* typhoid vaccinations if you live in an area where it is very prevalent. Three-yearly boosters are sufficient elsewhere.

What are the symptoms?

- High fever, usually not coming down to normal for several days.
- Persistent severe headache, general body aches and weakness.
- Diarrhoea (or constipation) with abdominal pain.
- Sometimes a rash of scattered red or pink spots on the trunk for a few days only.

What is the treatment?

If you have the above symptoms and signs you should be under the care of a doctor as soon as possible, and you would probably be admitted to hospital or have nursing care arranged for you. The best antibiotic is Chloramphenicol, which is very effective: except for eye infections and in special circumstances, this is the only illness for which chloramphenicol should be used.

YELLOW FEVER

What is it?

It is an acute feverish illness with jaundice caused by a virus that occurs in Africa and South and Central America.

How is it transmitted?

By the bite of an infected mosquito (Aedes aegypti, not the Anophelene which transmits malaria).

How can it be prevented?

Yellow fever vaccination gives protection for 10 years and should be given to everyone over 1 year old. Avoid mosquito bites: see *Malaria*.

What are the symptoms and signs of an attack?

Most cases are mild. The incubation period is 3–6 days, with sudden onset of high fever with headache, vomiting and muscle pains with severe exhaustion lasting 1–3 days. The temperature falls on the second to fifth days, with sweating, then may recur 3–9 days later with jaundice, the passage of protein in the urine and dark coloured vomit. In a severe attack the patient becomes progressively more ill, and needs to be under medical care, although there is no specific antibiotic which will cure this illness.

NOTE

A blood test should be done early in any sudden illness with high fever, to check for malaria.

7. PREGNANCY

Some people worry about being pregnant and going through a delivery, while others take it in their stride, feeling that pregnancy is, after all, a natural process.

Millions of babies each year are safely delivered and survive even where facilities are not good (witness the population explosion!). The following is not as detailed as a specialist book on pregnancy, but gives basic information and advice.

What is it?

A pregnancy occurs when a fertilized egg (or ovum) implants into the lining of the womb and starts to develop into a baby. The state of pregnancy continues until the baby is sufficiently developed to live outside the womb.

During the pregnancy the developing baby, inside its protective bag of fluid known as the amniotic sac, takes its nourishment directly from the mother's bloodstream through the placenta (also known as the afterbirth). This is an organ that develops with the baby, consisting mainly of the mother's and the baby's blood-vessels arranged in such a way that the bloodstreams are in close contact. Oxygen and nourishment are taken up by the baby, while waste products are passed out into the mother's blood.

Symptoms and signs of pregnancy

- The absence of the monthly period! In some cases, in the first couple of months after conception, there may be a small amount of blood-stained discharge at the time you would expect your period.
- Breast tenderness and swelling.
- Nausea, sometimes vomiting, usually in the morning.
- Frequency of passing urine.
- Weight gain or wider girth!
- The results of a pregnancy test, done at 42 days after the first day of your last normal period. It can be done later, but not earlier, on the first sample of urine you pass on the day of the test.

Some people feel tired and may be a bit 'up and down' emotionally; others feel better than ever before and look 'blooming'!

Miscarriage

If conditions are not quite right, or if there is something wrong with the developing baby (or foetus), the pregnancy may not go to completion, but end in a miscarriage. This means that the foetus, together with the placenta and the membranes, are expelled, usually with bleeding and spasmodic pain. The most common time for this to occur is when the foetus is between 6–12 weeks old. (See *Bleeding during pregnancy* for advice about what to do should this occur.)

ANTE-NATAL CARE

Why is it necessary?
This is basically undertaken to:
- Ensure the healthy growth of the baby.
- Ensure the mother remains healthy throughout the pregnancy.
- Spot any signs of developing problems as early as possible, and to deal with them appropriately.
- Prepare both the mother and the father for the delivery and for parenthood.

In some countries ante-natal care is given through a hospital clinic or a doctor's surgery. But it can be undertaken by any trained midwife or doctor with relevant (obstetric) experience, as long as they can get to laboratory facilities and can refer to an obstetric unit at the first signs of a problem developing.

Where there is an ante-natal clinic, attendance should start as soon as you know you are pregnant; the sooner investigations and check-ups can be done the better. In many countries women would attend the clinic, or see a doctor regularly, starting any time after the third month of pregnancy, at the following intervals:
- Up to 28 weeks, every 4 weeks.
- 28–36 weeks, every 2 weeks.
- 36–40 weeks, every week.

Pregnancy is usually counted in weeks and full term is 40 weeks.

What tests are done?
- Blood tests to check for anaemia and other problems.
- Blood pressure: if it is above 140/90, you need extra rest, and possibly hospital admission as the blood supply to the baby may be altered if the blood pressure is not controlled. Very high blood pressure may cause serious problems to mother and baby.
- Weight: this can also be done at home on the same scales every time. The total weight gain should be about 11kg/24lb or about ½kg/2.5lb per month.
- Urine: checked for protein, sugar or signs of infection.
- Size of womb and baby: by feel, and by ultra sound

scan (if available). One scan would be done at about 16 weeks when the baby is quite well developed. The heart can be seen, measuring about 1cm/½in across. Abnormalities of growth and development may show up. There is no clear evidence that ultrasound harms the baby. In some countries a test called amniocentesis is offered to mothers, especially if they are over 40 or if there is any history of congenital abnormalities in the family. A long needle is inserted carefully into the womb and some amniotic fluid withdrawn. This is studied under the microscope and chemically to ensure the baby is growing normally. There is a slight risk to the baby and should only be undertaken by fully trained personnel.

- Swelling of your ankles ('pitting oedema') and fingers: if combined with a rise in blood pressure and protein in the urine you will need to be admitted to hospital for bed-rest and special care.
- After the twenty-fourth week the baby's heart can be heard and will be listened for at each examination. There are also special instruments that can 'listen' to the heartbeat much earlier.

At some stage the size of your pelvis will be assessed, probably by vaginal examination, to see how easy it will be for the baby to be delivered normally. Towards the end of pregnancy the 'lie' of the baby is also important: is the head down, lying ready to enter the pelvis for its journey into the big wide world!

Of course, if any problems arise, these will be dealt with and other tests may need to be done, but these are the main points. There should be time for discussion about diet, breast-feeding and any problems or fears you may be experiencing.

BLEEDING DURING PREGNANCY

In the first 3 months a small amount of blood loss (like a discharge) may occur at the time you would expect your period. This, or other small amounts of bleeding, **needs bed-rest continued for 24 hours after the last bleed**. If there is any pain at all or if the bleeding becomes heavy or prolonged, then you should call the doctor as you may well be starting a miscarriage.

Avoid having sexual intercourse if there has been any bleeding.

Bleeding at any other time could be serious and must be assessed by a midwife or doctor as soon as possible, so do not delay calling one, or going straight to a hospital.

DIET DURING PREGNANCY

See also *Nutrition* in section 1.

Food

The general rules of a good balanced diet apply even more when you are pregnant. It is important that you provide your own body and the developing baby with all the nourishment required for growth: the baby takes what he or she needs from you, but you need to replenish the supply! Blood tests will show if you need iron and folic acid and you should take these if so advised. Avoid eating between meals, however, as you are likely to put on too much weight.

Should I take any drugs?

Avoid all medication if possible, although the *occasional* aspirin or paracetamol (if absolutely necessary) probably does little harm. Alcohol *does* do harm, as does smoking throughout pregnancy, so you should avoid both completely. Anti-malarials (except Maloprim or Fansidar) *must* be taken during pregnancy if you live in a malarious area; an attack of malaria can have very serious consequences. If you have to have antibiotics for some infection, make sure they are

of a type that are safe to take during pregnancy (see *Common drugs*, section 8). It is during the first 3 months that the developing foetus is most vulnerable, but care is needed throughout. There is some evidence (not clear as yet) that a multivitamin tablet a day protects the foetus in some way from developing certain abnormalities.

THE RHESUS FACTOR

It is important to know what blood group you are so that you can be given the correct blood should you need it. A small number of women are Rhesus negative; when they marry a Rhesus positive man, some of their babies may be affected by the mother's blood which may produce anti-bodies to the baby's blood (because they have different blood groups). A Rhesus negative woman should always have careful medical check-ups throughout pregnancy, and be given an Anti-D injection at once after delivery, or if she bleeds during pregnancy: the injection stops her developing harmful antibodies.

MINOR PROBLEMS

Nausea and vomiting

This is normally mild, and clears up in the third or fourth

month. However, if it is sufficiently severe to distress you or make you vomit frequently, there is safe treatment available, so ask for it. The nausea and vomiting are usually worse in the mornings, so it is usually called 'morning sickness'.

Back-ache

This tends to get worse as the baby becomes heavier. Be conscious of your posture; sit in straight-backed chairs rather than slouching in sofas, or put a pillow behind the small of your back if in a lower, softer chair. Your bed should be firm. Wear a good supporting bra as your breasts enlarge and become heavier.

Vaginal discharge

This tends to increase in pregnancy, especially in hot climates. It only needs treatment if you become sore or itchy or the discharge is offensive (see *Thrush* in section 5), but washing and showering more often will help. Do *not* use douches or Dettol: this only makes it worse.

Heart-burn

This tends to get worse as the baby grows and there is less room for your insides! Avoid spicy, very hot foods or drinks, and take antacids (these are safe) or milky drinks. It is sometimes better if you sleep and rest propped up rather than lying flat.

Odd aches and pains

● The womb contracts at odd times throughout pregnancy: this is not usually painful, but feels like a 'tightening' (known as Braxton Hicks contractions).
● Sometimes there can be a sharp 'stretching' pain at the side of the womb: this is probably because as it grows it stretches the ligaments around it.
● Leg cramps can be distressing at times: 'stretching' the relevant muscle by walking on it or pulling on the foot sometimes helps, or asking someone to rub the leg for you!

Fears and fancies

Fears are common and it is best to find someone you can talk to about them. Food fads are fine as long as they are not for alcohol or foods that are too fattening.

Sex during pregnancy

It is probably best to avoid it in the rather vulnerable period between the eighth and fourteenth week of pregnancy (which is when most miscarriages occur), but otherwise there is no need to do so, until the last month, when you may not feel much like it anyway. Many women are re-assured to know their husbands go on finding them attractive even in the later stages of pregnancy!

Constipation
This is common in pregnancy. The remedy lies in increasing your fluid and fibre intakes until you get the desired response. It is best to avoid laxatives. (See *Nutrition* in section 1.)

Excessive weight gain
As the baby grows you will, of course, put on weight. The amount varies, but a good overall average is about 11kg/24lb. The weight gain is higher towards the end, when it may be about 0.5kg/1lb per week, but anything above this needs watching. If your weight is going up very quickly you would need to consult a doctor about it. Weight gain is due to the baby's growth, but also (among other things) to an increase in the volume of fluid in the body, and if this is excessive it could cause problems.

Teeth
Have a dental check-up and ensure that any necessary fillings are done: decaying teeth can be a source of infection. You may find that your gums bleed more easily than usual, but do not let this deter you from cleaning your teeth.

Flying during pregnancy
Airlines will accept you up until 32 weeks. After this you will need a doctor's certificate to say you are unlikely to go into labour during the flight and giving the expected date of delivery. They would not take you after 38 weeks.

PREPARATION FOR LABOUR AND DELIVERY

If you are going into hospital
- Make sure you know exactly where you are to go and who you should contact at any time of day or night.
- Ensure that you have at hand everything you want to take with you ready packed: this means clothes for yourself and the baby, as well as other things like books, writing paper and so on.

If you are living in a country other than your own
- Find out where you have to register the nationality of the baby.
- Do you know and trust the midwife or obstetrician?
- Does the nearby hospital have facilities for blood transfusion, Caesarean section, forceps or vacuum deliveries, and resuscitating the baby?

- Make sure you have a 'life-line' to someone who can advise you when you come home again: about feeding, about nappy rashes, about a baby who is driving you to distraction because she or he won't stop crying! And all the 101 things you'll think of and wish you'd asked about.

Engagement of the head

This occurs at about 36 weeks in a first pregnancy, later in second or subsequent pregnancies. It means that the widest part of the baby's head passes into the bony circle of the mother's pelvis and stays there. You feel this as a 'lightening' of the load: the height of the womb drops a bit and you have slightly more space to breathe! It is a sign that all is well and proceeding normally.

The 'show'

Just before labour starts the neck of the womb (cervix) becomes soft and begins to stretch and widen. A 'plug' of blood-stained mucus is lost when this happens, and is called 'the show'.

'Breaking the waters'

This occurs when the bag of water in which the baby floats breaks. This can happen before true labour starts or after it has been established.

If it happens *before* labour starts you will experience a sudden loss of fluid that continues to leak in large or small quantities from the vagina. See your doctor or midwife at once for examination: if labour does not start soon after you may need to be started on antibiotics.

Usually, however, the membranes rupture some time after the contractions have started. Rupturing the membranes artificially is one way of inducing labour when a baby is taking its time coming or there is some other reason to get labour started.

LABOUR

This consists of the regular, strong contractions of the womb which eventually lead to the birth of the baby. It is said to be established when the contractions are coming at regular and increasingly frequent intervals. You can 'help' the process by learning (beforehand) to relax 'into' the contraction, to breathe properly (long, slow, controlled breaths) during the contraction and to relax completely to keep up your strength after each contraction. Your husband can be a great help here if he understands what is happening and stays with you to give moral (and physical) support.

The first stage

This lasts until the neck of the womb (cervix) is fully enlarged or dilated and ready for the baby to pass through. This may take 12–18 hours in a first pregnancy, so ensure you have something to occupy you, and some light food and frequent small drinks. In some, and usually in second or subsequent pregnancies, this stage may be as short as 3–4 hours.

The second stage

This lasts from full dilation of the cervix until the delivery of the child. This is usually only half an hour or less, but may be a bit longer in a first pregnancy. There is a strong urge to 'push' with each contraction. The doctor may make a small cut at the opening of the vagina (an episiotomy) at the end of this stage if the baby's head is likely to tear the tissues: a clean cut is easier to repair than a jagged tear!

When the baby is born

The baby should be given to the mother to hold immediately, if possible, and be put to the breast as soon as possible. Apart from the emotional 'bonding' this encourages, it also helps in expelling the placenta.

The third stage

This is the delivery of the afterbirth (placenta).

Throughout all this time everyone can work as a team to achieve as normal and safe a delivery as possible for both mother and baby, with good memories to look back on. The safety of the baby and of the mother must be the doctor's *first* consideration, of course.

After delivery

There will be a dark, blood-stained discharge (the lochia) that gradually becomes pale pink and disappears over about 4–6 weeks after delivery. If it remains bright red, or you start losing more heavily, perhaps with clots, or with an offensive smell, you should ask for a medical examination in case it has become infected.

Occasionally a small fragment of the placenta remains inside the womb, preventing it from returning to its normal size (involuting) properly. This will also lead to more bleeding and perhaps infection, so if you are concerned that all does not seem to be settling down normally, arrange to have a full internal examination. You should be having this routinely, in any case, at 6 weeks.

IF THERE IS NO DOCTOR OR NURSE PRESENT

Ensure you have the following ready:

- Clean boiled water.
- Sterile scissors or knife: boil in water or pass through a flame several times.
- Two pieces of sterile thread: boil these with the scissors.
- Place scissors and threads on a clean towel, ready for use. Get together a pile of clean cotton wool or squares of material.
- Another clean towel to receive and wrap the baby in: the baby will be very slippery and will need to be kept warm.

Before delivery

- Place mother comfortably on a clean sheet or large towel, with 2 or 3 pillows for her head if she is lying on her back. She can squat if she prefers.
- Wash your hands thoroughly in soapy water (use a brush for your nails if available) and rinse off.

During delivery

- Encourage the mother to push downwards into the vaginal area *only* if she feels a strong urge with each contraction. Her legs should be separated and bent upwards while she pulls on them from behind or around the knees to help the pushing.
- Wash the mother's vaginal area with soapy water, or a mild antiseptic solution.
- Between contractions, encourage the mother to relax completely, taking steady, long breaths, and to have a sip of water.
- As the baby's head parts the lips of the vagina, put your hand firmly on it to control its delivery, pushing gently downwards.
- As it emerges, feel around the baby's neck to make sure the cord is not around it. If it is, pull it gently and steadily over the head to release it. Do not jerk or pull too hard in case it breaks. If the cord will not come, you may have to tie the 2 threads tightly in 2 places around the cord and cut between them, then continue to deliver the baby.
- There will probably be a pause between the head emerging and the next contraction. Wait, use the cotton wool to clear the baby's mouth and nose of mucus.
- Have the towel ready to receive the baby.
- As the shoulders emerge (which may be with a rush) receive the baby into the towel and lift it straight onto the mother's tummy. Clear mucus from its mouth and

'flick' its feet to encourage it to cry.

- Leave the baby there while you deal with the cord. Feel for pulsations in the cord and 'milk' it towards the baby to empty as much blood into the baby as possible.
- When the pulsations cease, tie the two threads tightly around the cord about 2.5cm/1in apart, and about 7.5cm/3in from the baby. Cut between the two ties.
- Put the baby to the mother's breast and encourage it to suck. This will cause the womb to contract and start the process of delivering the afterbirth.
- The separation of the afterbirth may take 15–20 minutes. Do *not* pull on the cord other than very gently. When it has separated, it will be expelled into the vagina, and can be easily pulled out.

Emergencies

- If there is a lot of fresh bleeding, or the afterbirth does not separate after 30 minutes, you must take the mother as quickly as possible to the nearest hospital.
- If the baby does not start breathing within 30–60 seconds, clear the mouth of mucus and blood and pull the head back gently to lift the chin. Place your own

lips over the nose and mouth of the baby and puff gently into the baby's lungs. You should be able to see the chest rising as the air enters. Repeat this about 12–15 times per minute, taking a breath between puffs yourself. Remember the baby's lungs are delicate.

After one minute check for a heartbeat by feeling the left side of the chest with the flat part of your fingers. If you feel no heartbeat, place 2 fingers near the nipple, and press downwards firmly 5–6 times, with a sharp movement, but again remember the baby's ribs are fairly soft. Continue alternating mouth-to-mouth respiration and cardiac massage until the baby starts breathing spontaneously. Take the baby and the mother to hospital as quickly as possible for any further treatment that may be necessary.

WHEN YOU GET HOME AGAIN

Care of the breasts

When the baby sucks milk, the stimulation of the nipple causes a reflex increase in the milk flow. It is important to maintain this flow by regular breast-feeding. If the breast is left for too long (more than 4 – 6 hours) it will begin to fill with milk, there will be swelling and pain, and some blockage to the milk flowing towards the nipple. The chances of an infection occurring are then greater than when the milk flow is encouraged and maintained.

The breasts should be completely emptied at each feed, and you should learn to 'express' any milk that is left to ensure this and to prevent engorgement. Store this milk in a fridge for up to 24 hours (see hints for successful breast-feeding). If part of the breast becomes hard, painful and red, there may be infection developing: see a doctor as quickly as possible. You can start treatment at once by:

- Applying a flannel soaked in hot water for 10 minutes.
- Expressing milk.
- 'Stroking' the affected area down towards the nipple.

Repeat this hourly, or continuously, until you have been examined and advised about treatment.

You should ask for advice from a midwife or doctor if you have any difficulties with the breasts or nipples.

Feeding

'Breast is best' is actually true, and breast-feeding is strongly recommended for the following reasons:

- It is natural and hygienic, as well as cheap!
- Breast milk contains all the nutrients the baby needs for growth in the first few months.
- Breast milk gives some protection against infections, as antibodies from the mother are passed into the milk. It may also protect, to some extent, against the development of allergic conditions, such as asthma, eczema and some digestive problems.
- Breast-feeding creates a deep bond between mother and baby, and increases the baby's sense of security.
- Breast-feeding encourages the womb to contract, and you may be aware that you have cramps (like period pains) during breast-feeding.
- Breast-feeding should be continued for as long as both you and the baby enjoy it, but after 6 months the baby will need less from the breast and want more of other foods.

Hints for successful breast-feeding

- Most babies are happy on 3 – 4 hourly feeds, but there is no need to stick to a rigid routine. Demand feeding will soon settle into a pattern that is acceptable and will probably work out

into a fairly regular routine.
- Empty breasts completely at each feed. If the baby does not take all the milk, empty the breast by expressing the milk yourself, and store it in the fridge where it will keep for 24 hours or so. Use it to feed the baby another time; for example, in the middle of the night, when the father can take a turn to feed the baby from a bottle with the stored breastmilk.
- Remember, the more your baby suckles at the breast the better the stimulation to milk production.
- Do not worry about under or over feeding the baby: he will take as much as he needs (unless he is obviously ill and having difficulty in suckling).
- You will need to eat a good nourishing diet and plenty of fluids in order to maintain the milk supply. Do *not* try to lose weight until you have stopped breast-feeding. (See *Nutrition*, section 1.1.)
- You should *not* avoid foods, other than hot, spicy things, coffee, alcohol, and any foods you notice upset the baby (grapes or acidy fruits may sometimes cause diarrhoea in the baby). Some medicines will enter the breast milk, and you should check with the doctor if it is likely to cause any problems.

BOTTLE-FEEDING

Some women do have genuine problems with breast-feeding, and obviously bottle-feeding is a boon for them. It can be successful, given care with hygiene and the correct mixing of the formula. The advertising for bottle-feeds has led to many believing that bottle-feeding is better for the baby and more sophisticated than breast-feeding, but this is not true. There have been many tragic deaths as a result of unhygienic and incorrectly mixed bottle-feeds.

THE CONTINUING HEALTH AND GROWTH OF THE BABY

Mothers often worry that their baby is not 'getting enough' milk or that something is dreadfully wrong with a baby who cries a lot, or sleeps a lot! (Read also *Excessive crying in babies* and *Colic in babies* in section 5.4.) Remember that babies are actually tough little creatures in spite of their apparent fragility. They like to be handled gently but firmly, and to feel held and cuddled securely. The only way a baby has of communicating at the beginning is by crying or making a noise: so listen and try to understand what he is trying to tell you. It's usually very simple: 'I'm wet', 'I'm hungry', 'I feel lonely', 'I'm uncomfortable' or 'Please notice me'!

Is the baby getting enough milk?

Ensure you are drinking plenty of fluids and eating well (see *Nutrition*, section 1.1). Keep a weight chart and weigh weekly, or monthly, and enter it on the chart.

At the same time, enter any illnesses he or she has had, and the 'milestones', such as the first smile, the first time he rolled over, or first time she sat up alone. This gives you a good pictorial view of how the baby is doing. If the weight remains static or falls, this usually means there is something wrong (diarrhoea or ear-infection, for example) and a check-up by a doctor or nurse would be a good idea.

Changing 'stools'

The baby's faeces will change during the first weeks of life: at first the stools are dark greeny-black, then they become pale yellow, and gradually darken to the normal brown. When the baby's feeds are changed (when weaning, for example) the colour and consistency will also change.

Care of the cord

Many mothers worry about this. Simply keep it clean and dry by washing it a couple of times a day with sterile water (or with a weak salt solution, or spirit and powdering with a sterile or mildly antiseptic powder such as sterzac). It will drop off between the fourth and tenth days, leaving a protruding 'tummy button' that will gradually 'draw inwards' during the first few months. **If the area becomes red or oozes pus, the baby may need antibiotics. Do not ignore this: if not treated it could lead to serious illness.**

COMMON PROBLEMS IN THE FIRST FEW WEEKS

Crying

This is the baby's normal way of communication until it becomes a bit more sophisticated. Most mothers soon learn to understand their baby's cry. See *Excessive crying in babies*, section 5.4.

Vomiting

This is usually of no significance as all babies vomit small amounts during or shortly after a feed. A small amount will often be brought up with 'the burp' or wind. You may need to adjust the volume and frequency of feeds to suit the size of the baby's stomach: smaller more frequent meals may help. You should consult your health visitor or doctor if the vomiting becomes copious and the baby is not well in some way.

Skin rashes

These are common. A reddish rash of fine spots or blotches is often the result of overheating and is known as prickly heat. This usually means the baby is too warmly dressed, especially if there is also sweating. A rash around the mouth, nose or cheeks is common when the baby is dribbling a lot, especially when it is teething.

Nappy rash

This is also very common. It may be the result of the contact between the baby's sensitive skin and a wet nappy: a wet nappy should be changed as quickly as possible. The urine when in contact with air, produces ammonia, and this irritates the skin.

Sometimes a nappy rash is caused by a thrush infection: this will need to be treated with Nystatin cream or other anti-fungal cream.

It will clear quickly if the baby is left without a nappy as much as possible, the bottom cleaned and dried thoroughly, and a soothing cream applied (or Nystatin if necessary).

Sticky eyes

See *Eye problems*, section 5.4.

Constipation

See section 5.4.

'THE BABY BLUES'

What is it?

Post-natal depression is very common for a week or two after the delivery. The hormones are all re-adjusting and in the process can leave you feeling very up and down emotionally (labile). You may burst into tears, suddenly, for no apparent reason, or because you feel a failure when you're not sure you're producing enough milk, or because some seemingly trivial thing has upset you. Don't worry — this will pass — but a husband who is sympathetic, doesn't argue, gives you an extra cuddle or two, and is prepared to cuddle the baby for a while and do the nappy-changing will be a great help.

When you are away from your parents, remember, too, that this is a time when you might be particularly homesick for your own mum, and you may desperately need to talk with another mother about the details of how you felt or feel, and the things you are worrying about. New dads should not feel excluded: however much they shared and cared, they can never quite *know* what it feels like to go through the labour and delivery; only another mother can know.

If it doesn't pass

This only happens

occasionally. If you become increasingly depressed and especially if you feel detached from the baby and increasingly unable to cope after a week or two, please ask for medical help. This is most important: don't leave it, hoping it will go away. It *might*, but it might also develop into something very serious and long-standing. Get help sooner rather than later. If necessary, insist on travelling to where help is available. Husbands may have to be firm about this.

HINTS FOR HOT CLIMATES

- Remember to give the baby extra fluids; 30–60ml/1–2 oz boiled water between feeds is a good idea. If there is any diarrhoea, the most important thing to remember is that the baby needs even more **extra** fluids to replace what is being lost in the diarrhoea or vomit. If necessary, use a teaspoon and give 2–3 teaspoons full every 5 minutes: this usually stops the vomiting and ensures the baby gets enough. (See *Diarrhoea*, section 5.4.)
- Remember also in hot climates that there is no need to wrap the baby up as in colder climates. The baby will sweat to keep the body temperature down: prickly heat will soon develop if he is wrapped up too warmly. A light covering is probably all that is necessary.
- Do use a mosquito net which protects from mosquitoes as well as other creepy crawlies!
- If the baby becomes constipated it usually means he needs more fluids. Add a further measure of boiled water between feeds. A teaspoon full of brown sugar added to the water also helps.
- Never leave a baby for more than a few minutes in direct sunlight. A baby's skin is very sensitive and he may burn or become overheated.
- Never leave a baby in a car alone, especially not in the sun. The inside of the car becomes very hot, and the baby will rapidly become overheated.

8. COMMON DRUGS

Some general rules

This information is given for guidance only, and is not intended to replace consultation with a doctor.

Some of the drugs mentioned are generally available at a chemist's, or at any general store; some are for use only if advised by a doctor; and some are highly dangerous and should never be taken without strict medical supervision.

Advice is given about dosages and side effects, and, where appropriate, warning is given about dangers. Take note of warnings given: you could cause yourself a lot of ill-health, or worse, if you disregard it. Modern drugs are powerful tools which are useful and sometimes life-saving, if used correctly, but they can

also be dangerous if used incorrectly or inappropriately. Ensure that you follow instructions about dosage carefully, and avoid alcohol, for example, if advised to do so. Always check for the expiry date and do not use the drug after the given time.

It is better to avoid mixtures of medicines as these often contain a variety of drugs: keep to simple remedies where possible. If you have to take more than one medicine, check that they are safe to mix with each other. If you are on regular medicine (for blood pressure, for example) prescribed by your doctor, do not stop taking this if you are given something else, but check that they are safe to take together.

DOSAGES IN CHILDREN

Under 1 year

Usually ¼ of the adult dose, but please check, especially in the first month of life, as some dosages are calculated according to body weight.

Between 1–5 years

½ adult dose.

Between 6–12 years

¾ adult dose.

Notes about common drugs and their use

ANTIBIOTIC EYE OINTMENTS AND DROPS FOR CONJUNCTIVITIS

See also *Conjunctivitis*, section 5.1.
If the discharge, pain and irritation does not clear up within 3 – 4 days of starting treatment, seek medical advice.

- Chloramphenicol eye ointment: apply inside the lower eyelid twice daily.
- Chloramphenicol eye drops: apply 4 times daily at least.
- Albucid eye ointment (sulphacetamide sodium): apply inside the lower eyelid twice daily.
- Albucid eye drops: apply 4 times daily at least.

ANTIBIOTIC EYE OINTMENTS AND DROPS FOR TRACHOMA

If the discharge, pain and irritation does not begin to clear up within 3 – 4 days of starting treatment, seek medical advice.

- Achromycin eye ointment (tetracycline): apply inside the lower eyelid twice daily.
- Achromycin eye drops: apply 4 times daily at least.

Treatment may have to be continued for 6 weeks.

ANTIBIOTIC SKIN PREPARATIONS

For infected boils or injuries:

- Fucidin (Fucidic Acid) ointment.
- Cicatrin (Neomycin/ Bacitracin) powder.

ANTISEPTIC PREPARATIONS

These are all useful for cleaning wounds but beware of allergic reactions:

- Gentian Violet Solution. Useful for treating or preventing skin infections, mouth ulcers, and for vaginal thrush (soak tip of tampon and insert, 3 times per day for 2 – 3 days if necessary), although the colour can be a problem.
- Chlorhexidine Solution (pHisoMED).
- Savlon, liquid or cream.
- TCP liquid.
- Dettol liquid.
- Betadine (c. Iodine).

COUGH MIXTURES

There are an enormous variety of cough mixtures, many of which do very little, except soothe the throat a little. Most contain a variety of ingredients.

It is best to stick to simple mixtures, or to make your own soothing hot drinks, such as hot lemon and honey, or hot milk with a teaspoon of honey and a pinch of ginger (powdered), or a hot herbal tea drink. Steam inhalations, with or without the addition of a decongestant such as Friar's Balsam, Karvol, eucalyptus oil, will often help to settle a bout of coughing. Sucking a throat lozenge or cough pastille will also help.

Expectorants

These are intended to loosen the dry sticky phlegm that sometimes 'clogs' up the air tubes; they do not soothe the cough, but rather make it easier to cough up the phlegm. Expectorants often contain a decongestant (such as pseudoephedrine) and guaiphensin, and sometimes an antihistamine (such as diphenhydramine). They may therefore cause drowsiness.

Suppressants

These are intended to suppress the cough reflex, and should only be used at night to allow you (or others in the household!) to sleep, as it is better to get rid of the phlegm in the air tubes. It is also useful for dry hacking or exhausting coughs. Suppressants often contain similar ingredients to expectorants, plus codeine or pholcodine, or dextro-methorphan, all of which are effective cough suppressants. They are also constipating, and may also cause drowsiness. Blood pressure may be raised by some of the ingredients of cough mixtures and it is best to ask the chemist or a doctor if you are on other medication to ensure that it is safe for you to mix the different medicines.

SOOTHING SKIN PREPARATIONS

For irritating rashes, mild sunburns, and similar conditions:
- Calamine lotion.
- Caladryl cream.
- Zinc oxide cream.

STEROID SKIN PREPARATIONS AND TABLETS

These are powerful drugs and should be used only in consultation with a doctor.

ANTI-WORM MEDICINES

Also known as anthelmintics, for hookworm and roundworm:
- Bephenium hydroxynaphthoate (Alcopar): adults and children above 2 years should take 1 sachet; under 2 years, ½ sachet.

For threadworm and roundworm:
- Piperazine hydrate (Antipar): tablets, elixir, granules, 4 tablets or 15ml for adults; under 2 years, 2–4ml; 2–4 years, 5ml or 1½ tablets; 5–12 years, 10ml or 3 tablets.
- Piperazine hydrate (Pripsen): tablets, elixir, granules (double dose for roundworm.) 1 sachet, for adults, repeated after 14 days; 3 months–1 year, ⅓ sachet; 1–6 years, ⅔ sachet; 6–12 years, as adult.

FOR THRUSH INFECTIONS

Oral:
- Nystatin suspension: ½–1ml into mouth after food or drinks.

Vaginal:
- Canesten (Clotrimazole). Available as pessaries and creams.
- Nystatin. Available as pessaries and creams.

There are several other preparations too.

ANTI-MALARIALS

See *Malaria*, section 6.

I. ANTACIDS:

Chemical name of drug	ALUMINIUM HYDROXIDE
Proprietary names	Aludrox Antacid Asilone Dijex Milk of Magnesia Mist. Mag. Trisil. Many other preparations.
Uses	To neutralize acid in the stomach, therefore for indigestion and peptic ulcers.
Adult dosage	As directed on packet: usually 1–2 tablets or 10ml after meals.
Common side effects	Depending on ingredients, dry mouth, dizziness, constipation and other problems with prolonged use.
Warnings	1. If symptoms persist you should see a doctor. 2. Some mixtures contain sodium: beware if you are on a low salt diet.

II. ANTI-ALLERGIC PREPARATIONS:

Antihistamines and sodium cromoglycate (Intal)

Uses	These reduce or stop the allergic response. They can be used as tablets, eye drops, nasal sprays, bronchial sprays or syrups.
Warnings	All antihistamines are likely to cause drowsiness, and alcohol should not be taken at the same time as this makes it worse. Beware of driving or using machinery.
Chemical name of drug	CHLORPHENIRAMINE MALEATE
Proprietary names	Piriton tablets and syrup.
Adult dosage	4mg, 8-hourly.
Common side effects	Drowsiness, dry mouth.
Chemical name of drug	MEBHYDROLIN
Proprietary names	Fabahistin tablets and syrup.
Adult Dosage	50mg tablets, 1–2, 8-hourly.
Common side effects	Drowsiness, dry mouth.
Chemical name of drug	PROMETHAZINE HYDROCHLORIDE
Proprietary names	Phenergan tablets and syrup.
Adult dosage	10mg tablets, 1–2, 12-hourly.
Common side effects	Drowsiness, dry mouth.
Warnings	Phenergan is likely to remain in the bloodstream for 12–24 hours.

Chemical name of drug	TRIPROLIDINE+PSEUDO-EPHEDRINE
Proprietary names	Actifed tablets and syrup.
Uses	Anti-allergic, decongestant.
Adult dosage	½ – 1 tablet or 5ml twice daily.
Common side effects	Dry mouth, drowsiness.

Chemical name of drug	ANTAZOLINE SULPHATE
Proprietary names	Otrivine-antistin eye and nose drops.
Adult dosage	1 – 2 drops 3 times daily.

Chemical name of drug	SODIUM CROMOGLYCATE
Proprietary names	Intal inhaler or Spinhaler.
Uses	For asthma. Used regularly to prevent attacks developing.
Adult dosage	Usually 2 puffs 2 – 4 times daily.
Common side effects	Tightening of air tubes as powder or mist first enters.
Warnings	Must be used regularly. Does not relieve an actual attack of asthma.

Chemical name of drug	SODIUM CROMOGLYCATE
Proprietary names	Opticrom.
Uses	Allergic eye irritation: to be used regularly.
Adult dosage	1 – 2 drops 3 – 4 times daily.
Warnings	Does not cause drowsiness.

III. ANTIBIOTICS:

General Notes

Uses	These are drugs that kill bacteria. They have **no** effect on viruses. Particular infections require specific antibiotics, as not all bacteria are sensitive to all antibiotics.
Warnings	Repeated or inadequate use of antibiotics leads to bacteria becoming resistant to the antibiotic. **Always complete the course.** Some people are allergic to certain antibiotics. If you know you are allergic to a specific one, always tell the doctor or nurse who is prescribing for you, and do not take it, as the reaction could be dangerous.
Chemical name of drug	PENICILLIN Tablets and syrup
Proprietary names	Penicillin V, Crystapen G, Penidural and many others
Uses	Tonsillitis, chest infections, ear infections (if over 5 years old), some skin infections. In Rheumatic Fever — prevention of relapses and to protect against other problems.
Adult dosage	250mg, 6-hourly for 5–7 days.
Common side effects	Sometimes causes diarrhoea.
Warnings	See above. If allergic rashes develop, stop and change to another antibiotic.
Chemical name of drug	PENICILLIN Injections
Uses	Gonorrhoea, syphilis, other severe bacterial infections.
Warnings	Should **always** be prescribed and given by a doctor, or by a nurse under doctor's supervision.

Chemical name of drug	AMPICILLIN and AMOXYCILLIN Tablets and syrup
Proprietary names	Penbritin, Amoxil
Uses	Ear infections (if under 5 years old), tonsillitis, chest infections, urinary infections
Adult dosage	250mg, 6-hourly for 5–7 days.
Common side effects	Diarrhoea.
Warnings	If allergic rashes develop stop and change to another antibiotic.

Chemical name of drug	OXYTETRACYCLINE and TETRACYCLINE Tablets and capsules
Proprietary names	Oxytetracycline, Terramycin, Doxycycline, Minocin
Uses	Skin infections, chest infections, acne.
Adult dosage	Usually 250mg, 6-hourly, 5–7 days. Acne: 250mg, twice daily.
Common side effects	Metallic taste.
Warnings	Absorption decreased by milk and antacids. Do **not** give to children under 12 years, or in pregnancy, because it causes staining of teeth.

Chemical name of drug	CO-TRIMOXAZOLE (SULPHAMETHOXAZOLE+ TRIMETHOPRIM)
Proprietary names	Septrin and Septrin Forte Bactrim, tablets and paediatric suspension
Uses	Urinary tract infections (such as cystitis, kidney infections), sinusitis, some Salmonella infections. Alternative to Penicillin in cases of allergy.

Adult dosage	2 tablets, 12-hourly. Forte tablets are the equivalent of 2, therefore take 1 only per dose for 5–7 days, or 10 days for urinary tract infections.
Common side effects	Nausea, vomiting occasionally:
Warnings	If rash develops stop medication and change to other antibiotic if necessary. Do **not** give in pregnancy or to infants under 6 weeks.
Chemical name of drug	ERYTHROMYCIN Tablets and syrup
Proprietary names	Erythroped, Erythrocin
Uses	As an alternative to Penicillin, if allergic.
Adult dosage	250–500mg, 6–12 hourly, for 5–7 days.
Warnings	If rash develops stop medication and change to alternative, if necessary.
Chemical name of drug	CEPHALEXINS AND CEPHALOSPORINS
Proprietary names	Keflex, Ceporex
Uses	Good alternative to Penicillin. Useful for urinary infections.
Adult dosage	250–500mg, 8–12 hourly, for 5–7 days.
Warnings	As for 5 above.
Chemical name of drug	METRONIDAZOLE AND TINIDAZOLE
Proprietary names	Flagyl, Fasigyn
Uses	Amoebiasis, giardiasis, trichomonas vaginalis.
Adult dosage	*Flagyl:* 200–400mg, 8-hourly; for 7 days. *Fasigyn:* 4×500mg tablets at once, then 2 daily for 5–6 days.

Common side effects	Nausea, vomiting. Metallic taste.
Warnings	Do **not** use in pregnancy. Do **not** drink alcohol at same time: it will cause severe nausea and vomiting.
Chemical name of drug	CHLORAMPHENICOL
Uses	Only for typhoid or in eyedrops or ointments.
Adult dosage	NB A very powerful antibiotic, *dangerous* if used in children, and in the wrong situations; therefore should only be taken under medical supervision.

IV. ANTI-DIARRHOEALS:

Note:	The most important rule to remember in case of diarrhoea is: **replace lost fluids**, by drinking small and frequent amounts of fluid.
Chemical name of drug	KAOLIN MIXTURE, with or without small amounts of Morphine or Codeine
Proprietary names	Kaolin and Morphine Kaopectate, Kaodene
Uses	In profuse watery diarrhoea to thicken the stool; with Morphine or Codeine it reduces irritability and activity of the gut.
Adult dosage	5–10ml after each stool.
Common side effects	Constipation.
Warnings	Morphine and Codeine are constipating if continued for longer than necessary.
Chemical name of drug	ANTISPASMODICS, Tablets, syrups, or injections
Proprietary names	Imodium Capsules, Lomotil tablets or liquid and many others

Uses	Relaxes the muscle in the gut thereby reducing activity.
Adult dosage	*Imodium:* 2 capsules initially, then 1 after every stool. *Lomotil:* 4 tablets or 20ml initially, then 2 tablets or 10ml 6-hourly till diarrhoea stops.
Common side effects	Constipation, dry mouth, blurred vision, dizziness.
Warnings	Beware of using long term. If diarrhoea persists beyond 36–48 hours, seek medical help.

Chemical name of drug	ORAL REHYDRATION SOLUTIONS

Proprietary names	Rehidrat, Dioralyte Oralyte
Uses	Mixtures of salts and sugar accurately measured to replace what is lost by diarrhoea.
Dosage	Mix as directed with water, feed to child in small frequent doses and after every stool. Very good for children, especially babies, but expensive. (See *Diarrhoea* for alternative method.)

V. LAXATIVES:

Note	It is much better to eat a high fibre diet (see *Nutrition*) than to take laxatives. If you have become constipated, take 1–2 large tablespoonsful of bran, mixed with milk and cereal, yoghurt, soup, gravy or any other liquid, once or twice daily, until relieved. Drink plenty of liquids, and adjust your intake of bran and fibre until you can open your bowels comfortably and regularly. There will be some initial wind and abdominal discomfort.

Chemical name of drug	In emergency: GLYCEROL SUPPOSITORIES
Uses	Severe constipation causing pain and blockage at the anus or rectum.

Adult dosage	Insert 1 or 2 with gloved finger, and lie down for ½ – 1 hour.
Warnings	If problems continue you may need an examination and an enema.

Chemical name of drug	BISACODYL SUPPOSITORIES
Proprietary name	Dulcolax
Uses	Severe constipation causing pain and blockage at the anus or rectum.
Adult dosage	Insert 1 or 2 with gloved finger, and lie down for ½ – 1 hour.

Chemical name of drug	SENNA AND BISACODYL
Proprietary names	Senokot, Dulcolax tablets
Uses	Severe habitual constipation where the above measures do not help.
Adult dosage	1 – 2 tablets daily.
Warnings	If problems persist, consult a doctor.

Chemical name of drug	LACTULOSE
Proprietary names	Duphalac syrup
Uses	Severe habitual constipation where the above measures do not help.
Adult dosage	10 – 30ml daily.
Warnings	If problems persist, consult a doctor.

VI. PAIN-KILLING and ANTI-INFLAMMATORY DRUGS:

Chemical name of drug	ASPIRIN (300mg) or ACETYLSALICYLIC ACID
Proprietary names	Disprin, Aspro and many others, some with Caffeine (Soluble varieties are absorbed more quickly and are less irritant)
Uses	Headaches, sore throats, general aches and pains, earache, fever (reduces it and causes sweating).
Adult dosage	300mg tablets, 2 taken 4-hourly.
Common side effects	Irritation of stomach. Tinnitus (high-pitched noise in ears).
Warnings	Stop taking if these occur. Can cause bleeding from the gut. Dangerous in overdose.
Chemical name of drug	PARACETAMOL Tablets, capsules and syrup
Proprietary names	Calpol and many others.
Uses	General aches and pains, headaches, period pains
Adult dosage	500mg tablets, 1–2, 4-hourly.
Warnings	Overdose can cause liver damage.
Chemical name of drug	PARACETAMOL WITH CODEINE
Proprietary names	Panadeine Co., Parahypon, Paracodol and many others (some with Caffeine)
Uses	More severe pains than the above.
Adult dosage	1–2 tablets, 6-hourly.
Common side effects	Constipation.
Warnings	Overdose can cause liver damage.

Chemical name of drug	DIHYDROCODEINE TARTRATE
Proprietary names	DF 118
Uses	Strong pain-killers, also cough suppressant.
Adult dosage	1 – 2 tablets, 8-hourly.
Common side effects	Constipation.
Warnings	Addictive if taken regularly.
Chemical name of drug	IBUPROFEN
Proprietary names	Brufen, Nurofen
Uses	Anti-inflammatory for arthritis, pain-killing, period pains (for this, start taking 2 – 3 days before period starts, if possible).
Adult dosage	200 – 400mg, 8-hourly.
Common side effects	Nausea, stomach irritation.
Chemical name of drug	MEFENAMIC ACID
Proprietary names	Ponstan
Uses	As 5 above. Very effective for period pains if taken 2 – 3 days before period starts.
Adult dosage	250 – 500mg, 8-hourly.
Common side effects	Stomach irritation.

Chemical name of drug	NAPROXEN
Proprietary names	Naprosyn
Uses	As 5 above. Very effective for period pains if taken 2–3 days before period starts.
Adult dosage	250–500mg, 12-hourly.
Note:	PHENYLBUTAZONE, INDOMETHACIN are sold under many proprietary names, and are very effective anti-inflammatory, pain-killing drugs, but they cause blood problems which can be dangerous. There are many other pain-killers and anti-inflammatory drugs.

VII. SLEEPING TABLETS and TRANQUILLIZERS:
a) *SLEEPING TABLETS:*

Warnings	It is best not to get used to taking sleeping tablets every night. They can all cause dependence or addiction.
Chemical name of drug	NITRAZEPAM
Proprietary names	Mogadon
Uses	Insomnia. Effects last 12–24 hours or more. Should not be taken regularly.
Adult dosage	5–10mg at night.
Common side effects	Hangover, depression, nightmares.
Chemical name of drug	FLURAZEPAM
Proprietary names	Dalmane
Uses	As above.

Adult dosage	15–30mg at night.
Common side effects	Hangover, effect lasts into next day.
Chemical name of drug	TEMAZEPAM
Proprietary names	Euhypnos, Normison
Uses	Insomnia, effects last 6–8 hours: useful drug, does not cause hangover.
Adult dosage	10–30mg at night.
Common side effects	Few side effects or addictive qualities.

b) *TRANQUILLIZERS:*

Warnings	Depression can be unmasked by taking tranquillizers. All are addictive, especially Diazepam and Lorezapam.
Chemical name of drug	DIAZEPAM
Proprietary names	Valium, Calmpose
Uses	Tension, anxiety, insomnia.
Adult dosage	2–5mg, 8-hourly or at night.
Common side effects	Lightheadedness, confusion, depression.
Chemical name of drug	LORAZEPAM
Proprietary names	Ativan
Uses	Tension, anxiety, insomnia.
Adult dosage	1mg or 2.5mg, 8-hourly, or at night.
Common side effects	As above.

Chemical name of drug	CLOBAZAM
Proprietary names	Frisium
Uses	Tension, anxiety, insomnia.
Adult dosage	10mg, 8-hourly, or 1–2 capsules at night.
Common side effects	Few side effects and shorter acting than the above.
Warnings	Less addictive.

Warning	**Do not take barbiturates:** they are highly addictive and should only be used for specific problems such as epilepsy.

NATURAL REMEDIES

Many plants contain chemicals which have been extracted to make medicines and drugs. Many are useful in their natural form. One example of this is the papaya (or pawpaw) fruit, which contains an enzyme called papain which is often used for tenderizing meat. This same enzyme is very useful for treating wounds. The inside of the skin can be used as a dressing for the infected area as it will help to get rid of the pus and debris and promote healing. Papaya fruit also contain a high level of vitamin A (see *Nutrition*) and is therefore effective in preventing blindness caused by vitamin A deficiency.

9. COMPLEMENTARY HEALTH CARE SYSTEMS

The Holistic Approach

This approach sees a human being as a whole: he or she has physical, mental and spiritual needs, a particular personality or character, and is set within an environment and in relationship with others.

Illnesses or diseases are seen as the product of a combination of these factors, or the result of disharmony between them. In assessing the needs of the patient, all these factors are said to be taken into account by those who practise this particular type of therapy.

The holistic approach is not only to be found in the traditional or complementary systems of health care: many doctors and therapists using allopathic (or western) medicine are concerned with the whole person, and would keep all these aspects in mind while assessing a patient and his problem. More and more doctors expect their patients to take a personal responsibility for themselves and to be fully involved in all decisions about therapy. They recognize that many illnesses are caused by a person breaking the basic natural laws of healthy living, and require informed and well-motivated changes in attitude and life-style in order to achieve healing and harmony.

The following is an introduction to some of the more common and well-known complementary health care systems. For fuller information, the relevant books, colleges and associations will have to be consulted.

9.1 HOMOEOPATHY

What is it?

Homoeopathy as a system of healing was developed during the eighteenth and nineteenth centuries by Dr Samuel Hahnemann (1755–1845). He observed that illnesses treated by substances which caused the same symptoms as the illness could be cured by giving minute doses of these substances. He claimed that 'like should be cured by like' (*Similia similibus curantur*). He discovered that by a process of shaking the diluted substance vigorously, its potency could be enhanced so that increasingly small but effective doses could be obtained by serial dilution. This process he called 'potentization'.

What does treatment involve?

The homoeopath examines the patient fully and then spends a considerable time assessing him and his symptoms in minute detail, as the remedy has to match the symptoms as closely as possible. The symptoms are seen as the body's reaction to the underlying problem, and the homoeopath aims to stimulate the body's natural healing capacities to overcome it. Since homoeopathy uses such minute doses and aims at stimulating the body's own natural resources, there are no risks in taking homoeopathic remedies. **Anyone wishing to try out the effect of homoeopathic remedies should check to see that advice has not already been given to seek urgent medical help before delaying with these**.

The following is taken from a list of useful homoeopathic home remedies for acute conditions, recommended by Dr R. A. F. Jack, MB, ChB, MRCGP, FPSMDH, FFHom. Please read the instructions first, and use the remedies as advised, bearing in mind the caution given above.

Instructions

These tablets, pills and granules listed are homoeopathic, similar to those used in homoeopathic hospitals. They have the following unique properties:

(a) They have a pleasant taste and can be sucked or chewed.

(b) They keep their strength for years without deteriorating or losing their power, if kept sealed in their bottles.

(c) They can be given to any age of person, adult or child — even tablets to a baby, if the tablet is first crushed into powder. A convenient way to do this is to crush the tablet between 2 folds of clean grease-proof paper, or 2 dessert spoons. It doesn't matter if a few fragments fly off and are lost, there is still enough medicine left to work. The powder can then be given dry, or dissolved in water. *In acute conditions where frequent doses are needed, crush and dissolve 2 tablets (or 20 granules) in a cup of warm water, and give teaspoon doses of the water medicine, instead of a whole tablet. Being homoeopathic it will work just as well, and your supply will last longer.*

(d) They can be given to a child in its sleep: the child will simply rouse itself sufficiently to take the crushed tablet without properly waking. This is very useful when a child is found to be getting feverish after it has gone to bed.

(e) They are not poisonous — a baby could eat the contents of a whole bottle at once and would not be harmed — yet, for all that, they work in sickness, when the right medicine is given.

(f) Homoeopathic medicines do not interfere with other medicines, which can also be taken if necessary; but they are usually inactivated by substances containing Camphor, Eucalyptus or Menthol.

(g) They can safely be taken in any stage of pregnancy with no harmful effects either to the mother or the unborn baby.

(h) If in doubt as to which fever medicine to use, try No. 1, and if after 2 doses there is no improvement, try No. 2. It is like trying to open a locked door when you have 2 keys; you try the first, and if it does not fit, you use the second. So with all these medicines, if the first does not work, you have done no harm, but only wasted it. You can then try a different one, as long as the instructions on the label seem to match the patient's symptoms.

Useful homoeopathic home remedies for acute conditions

ACONITE:

SHOCK and No. 1 FEVER:

For shock, croup, effects of fright or chills; any emergencies, such as accident, animal bites, asthma, haemorrhage, bereavement, fear, distress, breathlessness, palpitations, tremblings, or numb tinglings. At onset of fevers, if thirsty, restless, anxious.

10 granules (1 tablet or pill) ¼-hourly until relief.

ANT. CRUD.:

No. 2 STOMACH:

When cross, touchy, depressed. When baby vomits feeds, white-coated tongue, corners of mouth cracked. No appetite. Sick headaches from catarrh, alcohol, bathing. Wants sharp drinks, or pickles. Belching, bloated.

10 granules (1 tablet or pill) ¼-hourly until relief.

ANT. TART.: **No. 2 COUGH:**

When touchy, drowsy, very weak. Cold, clammy sweat; pale or bluish face, white-coated tongue. Breathless, suffocating, gasping; must sit up. Rattling cough, unable to expectorate. Worse for warmth.

10 granules (1 tablet or pill) ¼-hourly until relief.

ARNICA: **INJURY:**

For bruises, sprains, concussion, crushed fingers, road accidents, etc. If shocked, give Aconite first.

Also for exhaustion, or muscle aching (heart, chest, back or limbs) from strain, sport or overuse. Use before and after dental surgery.
10 granules (1 tablet or pill) 2-hourly until relief.

ARS. ALB: **SICKNESS and DIARRHOEA:**
When sickness and diarrhoea simultaneously (?gastric 'flu, ?food poisoning), feeling very cold, anxious, exhausted, can't rest. Burning pains in stomach. Thirst for warm drinks. Can't bear sight, smell of food.
10 granules ¼-hourly until relief.

BELLADONNA: **EARACHE and No. 2 FEVER:**
When burning hot, flushed, wide-eyed, excited (?delirious, ?scarlet rash). Thirsty but won't drink. Also sore throats, colic, throbbing headaches, throbbing boils, severe earache with above symptoms. Effects of sunstroke.
10 granules (1 tablet or pill) ¼-hourly until relief.

BRYONIA: **PAIN or HEADACHE:**
For bursting headaches, migraine, arthritis, pleurisy, only when pains worse from movement, breathing, warmth; better for pressure, lying quiet, keeping still in cool. Irritable, parched, thirst for cold drinks.
10 granules (1 tablet or pill) 4-hourly until relief.

CAMPHOR: **CHILL:**
When icy cold following chill. First stage of cold, when chilled, sneezing, better for warmth. Onset diarrhoea from chill, if feeling 'frozen'.
10 granules (1 tablet or pill) every 5 minutes, until relief and feeling warm. Keep bottle separate. Camphor vapour inactivates other homoeopathic medicines.

CANTHARIS: **BLADDER and BURN:**
Cystitis when urine scalds, passed drop by drop. Unbearable urging and frequency. Also burns and scalds, better for cold applications. Also burning, itching blisters (erysipelas). Gnat bites.
10 granules (1 tablet or pill) 2-hourly until relief.

CARBO VEG.: **WIND and COLLAPSE:**
When stomach distended, passing wind up (? and down), must sit up, loosen clothing. When collapsed, ? pale, ? bluish, pulseless, cold, cold sweat, needs propping up, gasping, must have air and be fanned.
10 granules (1 tablet or pill) every 15 minutes until relief.

CHAMOMILLA: **FRANTIC PAIN:**
For unbearable pains; earache, toothache, teething, better being picked up, ? one cheek hot. Colic, diarrhoea, green motions. Bad tempered, impatient, worse for heat, anger.
10 granules every 5 minutes until relief.

COLOCYNTH: **COLIC:**
For agonizing colic, better doubling up, hard pressure, heat, twisting about. Griping pains causing distension, belching, vomiting, ? diarrhoea. Colic and neuralgia from anger or 'getting worked up'.
10 granules (1 tablet or pill) ¼-hourly until relief.

EUPHRASIA: **MEASLES and HAY FEVER:**
For onset measles when eyes streaming, tears burn, can't face light. Running nose, sneezing cough. Throbbing headache. Hay fever, as above, worse indoors, in warmth, evenings.
10 granules (1 tablet or pill) 2-hourly until relief.

GELSEMIUM: **INFLUENZA and 'NERVE':**
When hot, flushed, aching, trembling, dizzy, drowsy, feeling 'drugged' or weak. Headache, limbs and eyes feel heavy, back chilly. Sneezing, running nose. Sore throat, difficulty swallowing. No thirst. Also, upsets from 'nerves'.
10 granules (1 tablet or pill) 2-hourly until relief.

IPECAC: **NAUSEA and No. 1 COUGH:**
For persistent nausea, ? vomiting, with clean tongue, much saliva. Onset violent suffocating, wheezing bouts, coughing. Also nose bleeds, haemorrhages, with nausea.
10 granules (1 tablet or pill) 2-hourly until relief.

MERC. SOL.: **FEVERISH COLD:**
When feeling chilly in cold, hot in warmth, weak, trembling, offensive sweat and breath. Profuse greenish catarrh, salivation, thirst. Diarrhoea with persistent straining, slime, ? blood. All symptoms worse at night.
10 granules (1 tablet or pill) 2-hourly until relief.

NATRUM MUR.: **RECURRENT COLD and DEPRESSION:**
For 'sneezy' colds with fever blisters, if much nasal catarrh; if feeling cold, but worse in warm room. Greasy skin, likes salt, thirsty. Also depression, if irritable, weary, ? weepy (on doctor's advice, only).
10 granules (1 tablet or pill) 4-hourly until relief.

NUX VOM.: **STOMACH and No. 2 'FLU':**
When chilly, irritable, ? quarrelsome. Delayed indigestion, nausea, constipation, or frequent unsatisfactory bowel actions. Itching piles. 'Flu' or raw throat, if chilled when uncovered. Stuffy colds if worse in cold air. Infant's snuffles if irritable.
10 granules (1 tablet or pill) 4-hourly until relief.

PHOSPHORUS: **LARYNGITIS and REPEATED VOMITING:**
When chest tight, hoarse, hurts to talk, ? loss of voice. Dry, tickling, racking cough, worse in cold air, worse talking. Gastritis with craving for cold drinks,? vomited immediately.

Nervous. Thunder headaches.
10 granules (1 tablet or pill)
2-hourly until relief.

PULSATILLA: **CATARRH and No. 2 MEASLES:**
When thick, coloured catarrh, of eyelids or nose. Loss of smell. Dry mouth (no thirst). Better in open air. Catarrhal cough, worse warm room. Measles. Indigestion from fat, rich food.
10 granules (1 tablet or pill)
4-hourly until relief.

RHUS TOX.: **RHEUMATISM, ARTHRITIS:**
When pains, stiffness, worse in wet weather, cold air, in bed, after rest (first movements hurt). Better keeping moving. 'Flu', dry cough with above symptoms. Also itching blisters (? erysipelas, ? shingles) if restless. Tendon sprains.
10 granules (1 tablet or pill)
4-hourly until relief.

SULPHUR: **SULPHUR:**
For burning, itching skin rashes, worse for warmth, worse for scratching, washing, clothing. Burning boils, styes and piles. Hungry, easily fatigued, hot 'flushes', hot feet (uncovers them in bed). Morning diarrhoea.
10 granules (1 tablet or pill)
twice daily until relief.
Maximum 6.

9.2 NATUROPATHIC MEDICINE

What is it?
The British Naturopathic and Osteopathic Association claims that this is a complete system of healing, which 'seeks to promote health by stimulating and supporting the body's inherent power to regain harmony and balance'.

What does treatment involve?
The naturopathic practitioner sees his task as one of educating the patient 'to take more responsibility for his health, and to assist him to understand the fundamental laws of health relating to rest, exercise, nutrition and hygiene' . . . and also of 'using natural remedies to increase the vitality of the individual, and to remove any obstructions which may be interfering with the normal functioning of the body'.

Qualifications
An accredited naturopath has osteopathic training for 4 years, and also uses a variety of other treatments, such as dietetics, fasting, hydrotherapy, acupuncture, and education about natural

hygiene and the place of rest and exercise in the healing process. Many will see their work as complementary to that of the general practitioner, and will refer patients to an allopathic doctor if this is appropriate.

9.3 OSTEOPATHY

What is it?
The British Naturopathic and Osteopathic Association says that osteopathy is 'a system of healing that deals with the structure of the body, that is, the bones, joints, ligaments, tendons, muscles and general connective tissues and their relationship to each other.'

In 1874 Dr Andrew T. Still developed the philosophy and practice of osteopathy, based on the belief that 'the body is selfhealing, and that an uninterrupted nerve and blood supply to all the tissues of the body is indispensible to their normal function.' He worked out a system of manipulation intended to restore and re-align structures to the normal.

What do osteopaths treat?
They claim to be able to relieve or treat many types of back-ache, neck problems, headaches, migraines, asthma, constipation, period pains, heart disease and digestive problems. They do not claim to be able to cure all diseases by manipulation of the spine.

What does treatment involve?
The osteopath will take a detailed medical history and make a full examination, including X-Rays, blood or urine tests if necessary. Treatment will be by manipulation, but those who are also naturopaths will use other naturopathic methods, taking a holistic view of the patient.

Warning!
Go only to osteopaths who are registered, and have therefore had full training.

Qualifications
Members of the Register of Osteopaths are entitled to use the designation MRO after their names. They will have undergone a 4-year training course in osteopathy.

9.4 CHIROPRACTIC

What is it?

The British Chiropractors' Association defines Chiropractic as 'an independent branch of medicine concerned with the diagnosis and treatment of mechanical disorders of the joints, particularly spinal joints, and their effect on the nervous system. Diagnosis includes the use of X-Rays, and treatment is done mostly by hand, without the use of drugs or surgery.

What do chiropractors treat?

Chiropractors claim that slight malalignments (called 'subluxations') of the spinal vertebrae may cause joint and back problems, but also such things as migraine, dizziness, chest pains, and that correction by manipulation will relieve the problem.

What does treatment involve?

A chiropractor will take a full history, and examine the patient, including the posture. The treatment involves manipulation of a specific type, and may also include massage, pressure and heat treatments with general advice. Chiropractic manipulation is said to be very safe, and the risks of treatment are minimal.

Qualifications

Chiropractors who trained before 1969 will have done their training in the USA or Canada; since then many practitioners will be graduates of the Anglo-European College of Chiropractic, who are given a Diploma.

9.5 THE ALEXANDER AND FELDENKRAIS TECHNIQUES

What are they?

F. M. Alexander was an Australian who went to the UK at the turn of the twentieth century and taught a technique of restoring correct balance and poise to the way we use our bodies, and especially our posture. Alexander lessons are techniques of re-education, and require a series of at least 12 lessons under supervision of a teacher. It is claimed that applying the

Alexander techniques alters one's basic body image, and can help to alleviate depression and tension.

Moshe Feldenkrais used aspects of the Alexander technique and combined these with aspects of eastern body concepts and exercises. His technique for restoring full efficiency and function to the body is a series of exercises which increases awareness of body movements. It is especially popular in the USA.

9.6 ACUPUNCTURE AND CHINESE MEDICINE

What is Chinese Medicine?

Traditional Chinese Medicine is a complete and ancient system of healing dating back to at least 400–500BC, possibly earlier. It uses acupuncture, herbal remedies, diet and exercise, for the prevention and treatment of disease. It is based on the belief that life is activated by a vital life force or energy called *chi*, which pervades all of nature. Health is maintained by the free flow of *chi* through the body. The emphasis is on the prevention of disease and on maintenance of health through correct diet, lifestyle, and regular exercises designed to stimulate the free flow of *chi*.

Everything in life can be classified into 2 opposing but balanced forces known as *yin* and *yang*; disease implies an imbalance that has to be corrected. Alongside this is also a theory of 5 elements, and there is also a belief in the 'wholeness' of the human being: he is an indivisible unit made up of body, mind and spirit, inextricably linked with the environment. Illness comes from within man himself, or from the environment, and treatment is aimed at improving the patient's ability to cope with these factors. The quality of the person's *chi* is of the utmost importance to the outcome of the illness.

What is acupuncture?

Over the surface of the body is thought to run a network of meridians or channels along which energy can pass; the channels connect with the inner organs. The *chi* can be manipulated at certain points along the meridians, to stimulate or treat specific organs at distant sites: this is the practice of acupuncture. Diagnosis of a problem requires a thorough examination of the patient using a variety of techniques which include palpation of the pulses and examination of the tongue.

The treatment is aimed at the whole person, not just the symptom.

Interest has been growing in countries outside China in the subject of acupuncture and much research is being done. Some scientific understanding for its efficacy is being formed. Western influence has led to some modernization of techniques, and these techniques have been increasingly investigated and used in the West, where they are often isolated from the wider philosophy which lies behind their use in China. The use of acupuncture in anaesthesia and pain control has roused special interest, and in some countries this form of treatment is available in clinics for, for example, the relief of pain.

Warnings!
Acupuncture needles are made of stainless steel, and should always be sterilized between patients, or discarded if used on a patient with a history of hepatitis. When seeking treatment, ensure that the acupuncturist is properly qualified.

Qualifications
The following are the qualifications held by properly trained acupuncturists:
BAAR British Acupuncture Association & Register
RTCM Register of Traditional Chinese Medicine
TAS Traditional Acupuncture Association
Lic.Ac. B.Ac. D.Ac. British College of Acupuncture

9.7 HERBAL MEDICINE

What is it?
Plants and extracts of plants have been used in medicine for thousands of years in all parts of the world. Chinese medicine incorporates the use of herbal remedies, as do the Indian systems of Ayurveda and Unani. Many modern drugs used in allopathic medicine have been derived from plants.

The basis of modern herbalism is the belief that the whole plant is safer and better than the individual constituents derived from it, and that the patient should be treated as a whole. There has been some research, and more needs to be done, into herbal remedies. There seems to be some truth in the belief that certain medicinal substances cause less harm and are more effective if taken 'in their context', as part of the whole plant. However, dosages cannot be monitored accurately in the way that allopathic drug dosages can be.

Qualifications
A medical herbalist usually trains for 4 years. Students are taught by doctors, and their examinations are marked by doctors. They practise in much the same way as a General Practitioner would, and use similar diagnostic tools and methods. Some will refer to allopathic doctors if they feel the problem cannot be dealt with by them, and most will not interfere with treatment already started. They would use dietary advice and general health education as part of their treatment.

Herbalists usually fall into the following groups:
- The retail herbalists, supplying remedies across the counter.
- The Hakims: Indian herbalists.
- Chinese Herbalists: traditional Chinese or modern Europeans who combine herbalism with acupuncture.
- Medical Herbalists: these are usually members of the National Institute of Medical Herbalists.
- A miscellaneous group, using many methods such as radionics, hair analysis, iris diagnosis, and so on.

9.8 AYURVEDA, SIDDHA AND UNANI SYSTEMS

What are they?
These are the main Indian medical systems that have been well developed for at least 2,000 or 3,000 years. Ayurvedic Medicine is a complete system incorporating diagnosis and treatment of illnesses, and giving detailed instructions about health maintenance and life-style. The main Ayurvedic texts date back to the fifth and second centuries BC. They show that the system was well established, and used concepts and tools which are considered modern today, including an understanding of the spread of infections through pathogenic organisms!

Ayurveda is based on the belief that there needs to be a balance between all the energies and constituents of life. There are thought to be 5 basic elements (*doshas*) and 3 basic energies (*gunas*). The environment and food, as well as people, contain these forces in varying degrees, and all need to be balanced or in harmony to maintain good health.

Ayurvedic medicines are complicated herbal remedies specially made up for each patient, after an exhaustive assessment of the patient and all environmental factors surrounding him (including the astrological aspects). There are 8,000 medicines in the Ayurvedic system.

Unani medicine is derived from Ayurveda, with strong Greek and Arabic influences. The word *unani* is commonly used in Indian languages to indicate 'of Greek origin'.

Siddha is an offshoot from these systems, using minerals as the basis of medication. The word *siddha* is derived from a Sanskrit root meaning 'perfection' or 'completion'.

Unfortunately some potent Ayurvedic medicines used in the west contain poisonous amounts of heavy metals such as lead and mercury.

All these systems use also massage, diets, special exercises, surgery, blood-letting, and purification procedures.

9.9 SOME OTHER THERAPIES

ANTHROPOSOPHICAL MEDICINE
This is a well-established comprehensive system for treating ill-health, and is widely practised in Germany in particular. It is based on the philosophy of Rudolf Steiner (1861–1925), combining Ayurvedic beliefs with modern herbal remedies, homoeopathy, heat, cold, art and eurythmics.

AUTOGENIC TRAINING
This is a method of learning to use relaxation of the body as a means of gaining co-operation with the instincts and emotions to promote health and harmony. Practical formulas can be worked out to deal with common conditions and stressful situations. It is a method which has to be taught by trained practitioners.

BIOFEEDBACK
This is a system of learning how to become aware of and control body functions. It is possible to learn to lower blood pressure, warm cold hands, control migraines and other physical and mental problems. Sophisticated biofeedback machines have been developed which can measure levels of stress, using small body changes such as pulse rate and sweating.

REFLEXOLOGY or ZONE THERAPY

Chinese and Japanese medicine, and some other systems, believe that every organ has a corresponding situation on the hands, feet, face, ears and eyes. The Chinese and Japanese also have systems of massage based on such correspondences, and pressure points called *shiatsu*. These ideas have been developed and are being used in Zone Therapy in the USA, and the system is also becoming popular in other parts of the West.

GLOSSARY

acute sudden

allergy an exaggerated sensitivity reaction; usually takes the form of a rash or of swelling of eyelids or face; may also affect the eyes, nose, lungs and digestive system

bacteria minute organisms which may or may not cause illness; they are single-cell, and can only be viewed through the microscope

benign unlikely to cause death

cap a barrier method of contraception inserted into the vagina at the entrance to the womb before intercourse, and removed 6–8 hours afterwards

catheter a fine rubber tube

chronic ongoing, of long duration

compress several layers of material, often soaked in cold or hot water, ice, witch-hazel

condom a 'sheath' placed over the erect penis to prevent pregnancy

convulsion a sudden contraction of some or all the muscles; several such contractions may occur rhythmically as in an epileptic fit or in a febrile convulsion

decongestant a medicine or substance that reduces congestion of the breathing passages

dehydration a drying out of the tissues as a result of fluid being lost without being replenished, as, for example, in diarrhoea and vomiting

diaphragm also known as the dutch cap, a barrier method of contraception inserted into the vagina at the entrance to the womb before intercourse, and removed 6–8 hours afterwards

douche a stream of water directed into a body cavity in order to wash it out

embolism a blood-clot travelling round in the circulation

enzyme a ferment or substance that speeds up or encourages a chemical reaction to take place

excreta waste material from the body: urine or faeces

faeces waste material excreted by the bowel

febrile feverish

fibre-optic a tube of very fine glass fibres which transmit light and which can be used to view internal organs

haemorrhage severe heavy bleeding

incubation period the time between the first contact with an infectious illness and the development of the first signs of the illness

infection invasion of the body by organisms causing disease

insomnia disturbed sleep, or inability to sleep

intravenous into a vein

lesion an abnormal lump or patch

locally limited to one particular area

low-grade fever fever which does not go above about 38.5°C or 101°F

malaise feeling of ill-health

malignant any illness or growth likely to cause death

medication any medicine or drug used in treating an illness

menstrual anything relating to a woman's monthly periods or menstruation, thus, for example, pre-menstrual: occurring before a period

nausea a sensation of sickness, often preceding vomiting

obstetric related to the delivery of babies

orally by mouth

palpitations a sensation of the heart racing or beating irregularly

prophylaxis preventive measures or drugs taken to prevent an illness

respiratory relating to the breathing organs, that is, nose, wind-pipe (trachea) and lungs

sebaceous fatty, related to sebum, the fatty material produced by the sebaceous glands in the roots of the hairs

semen the secretion from the testicles; usually contains sperm

septic infected by pus-forming bacteria

sponge a circular sponge impregnated with spermicide which is inserted in the vagina to prevent conception

steroid a group of powerful drugs which reduce inflammation

suppository medicine contained in a solid cone which can be inserted into the rectum

thrombosis a clot of blood

ulcerate the process by which an ulcer is formed. An ulcer is an area of skin or organ lining which has broken down leaving a sore with an edge

virus an organism which is even smaller than bacteria and can only be seen through an electron-microscope and which may or may not cause disease if it enters the body

viral caused by a virus: for

example, a viral infection

vomit a sudden, uncontrollable reflex reaction of the food tube and the stomach which forces the food or contents of the stomach to be brought up through the mouth

x-rays short electro-magnetic waves which penetrate many tissues and are used to produce pictures of substances such as bone, which they are unable to penetrate

HOW TO USE A THERMOMETER

How does it work?

A thermometer uses the fact that mercury expands when warmed. A small amount of mercury is held in 'the bulb', which is made of a thin layer of glass. The bulb connects with a hollow tube encased in thick glass, which has markings on it. The thick glass acts as a magnifier. The markings are numbered in degrees Fahrenheit or Centigrade (or both). When the mercury in the bulb is warmed it expands and rises in the hollow tube. The level to which it rises depends on the heat (or temperature) surrounding it.

To prevent the column of mercury from falling back as it cools, a small kink is provided in the tube where it connects with the bulb. In order to reset the thermometer for a new reading, shake down the mercury to return it to the bulb once it has cooled. In hot climates it may be necessary to immerse the thermometer in cold water to enable this to be done effectively.

Where do I put it?

The thermometer may be used in several places:
- the armpit (axilla) or the groin
- the mouth
- the rectum

The mouth and the rectum will give the most accurate readings, but in small children it should never be placed in the mouth as they may bite and break it. Neither the glass nor the mercury will do them any good! For a child, the safest place is the armpit or the groin, or if he can be controlled, the rectum. Remember that the mouth temperature will be affected by cold or hot drinks taken within 10–15 minutes.

How to take a temperature
- Shake down the column of mercury to well below the 'normal' mark (37°C/98.4°F).
- Place the bulb of the thermometer and part of the shaft in the chosen place (under the tongue if in the mouth, with lips kept closed).

- Leave for ½ – 3 minutes —
  read the instructions with
  the thermometer.
- Take out, and read off the
  marking to which the
  mercury column has risen.

HOW TO TAKE A PULSE

What is a 'pulse'?

The pulse is the rise in
pressure that occurs
throughout all the arteries
when the heart beats
(contracts). It can be felt in
several places, using 2 or 3
fingertips placed over an
artery. The most common
places used are:

- At the wrist: this is the
  commonest place. Hold
  your hand with the palm
  facing you. Place 2 or 3
  fingertips just below the
  wrist joint in line with the
  thumb. You should be able
  to feel a regular pulse beat
  if you press down gently
  just to the outside of a
  tendon (which feels like a
  solid line running up from
  the wrist).
- Under the jaw: place your
  fingertips just below the jaw
  where it makes a curve up
  towards the ear. Press
  inwards gently, and you
  should be able to feel a
  fairly strong regular pulse
  beat.

Index